PARENTING HOMO SAPIENS

The 7 Eternal Truths
for Raising Happy Humans

DR KARISHMA STRETTON
BMedSci, LLB, MBBS

Parenting Homo Sapiens
Published by Impressum, Newcastle NSW

© Dr Karishma Stretton 2021
www.drkarishmastretton.com.au

Cover and internal design by Impressum www.impressum.com.au

National Library of Australia Cataloguing-in-Publication entry
Author: Stretton, Karishma
Title: Parenting Homo Sapiens / Karishma Stretton
ISBN: 978-1-922588-06-7 (paperback) | 978-1-922588-05-0 (ebook)

All rights reserved. No part of this publication may be reproduced, stored in, or introduced into a retrieval system, or transmitted, in any form, or by any means (electronic, mechanical, photocopying, recording or otherwise) without the prior written permission of the publisher.

"Conventional thought attributes the character and traits of our lives to be preprogrammed in the genes. However, the revolutionary field of epigenetics reveals that perceptions and behavioral programs derived from prenatal and childhood experiences define the character of our lives, controls our health, and even regulates gene expression. Limiting and disempowering beliefs acquired during this sensitive development period seriously undermine health and sabotage an individual's aspirations and desires.

An important contribution toward healing societal dysfunction and ensuring the healthy development of future generations is provided in PARENTING HOMO SAPIENS by Dr. Karishma Stretton. This highly readable book provides a valuable compilation of science, spirituality, and Dr. Stretton's personal insights derived from her experiences with patients, as well as with her own children. PARENTING HOMO SAPIENS is an important resource that illuminates how parental beliefs and emotions profoundly shape the lives of children, and as importantly, contributes to the nurturing of our evolving civilization."

Bruce H. Lipton, Ph.D., stem cell biologist, pioneer in epigenetic science, and author of the bestselling books *The Biology of Belief, Spontaneous Evolution* (with Steve Bhaerman) and *The Honeymoon Effect*.

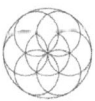

"Karishma brings a wealth of wisdom and experience, including as medical practitioner and mother, to this beautiful distillation of the essence of parenting. PARENTING HOMO SAPIENS reminds us that, as parents, we truly hold the future in our hands, and provides us with the biological understandings and practical tools that will support us to raise happy humans."

Dr Sarah Buckley MB, ChB. Dip Obst., author of the bestselling book *Gentle Birth, Gentle Mothering: A Doctor's Guide to Natural Childbirth and Gentle Early Parenting Choices.*

*To my family for always
illuminating my path*

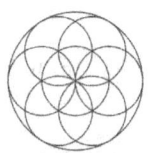

CONTENTS

INTRODUCTION *XI*

TRUTH ONE *1*
THE HUMAN FOETUS, BABY AND CHILD HAVE FUNDAMENTAL BIOLOGICAL EXPECTATIONS

    Biological Expectations... 1

    Attachment 6

    Attachment at Different Stages of the Parenting Journey.................. 11

    Conception and Pregnancy 12

    Birth - Bringing Human Consciousness into this World................. 18

    The First Moments After Birth.. 36

    Continuation of Bonding and Attachment 39

    Striving to Meet Human Potential...................................... 47

TRUTH TWO *50*
WHAT WE INSCRIBE IN THE CHILD'S MIND WILL ECHO THROUGHOUT THEIR LIFETIME

    Sowing the Seeds of Change.. 50

    Shifting Focus 51

    Nourishing the Brain With Love 55

    Rapid Download 61

    Door to the Subconscious Mind 64

TRUTH THREE — 67
PARENTS ARE GENETIC ENGINEERS – EPIGENETICS AND ENGINEERING THE FUTURE

- Epigenetics 67
- Epigenetics as a Reason to Honour Child Creation 68
- Trans-generational Inheritance of Epigenetic Markers 73
- Genes and Human Behaviour 73
- Epigenetics as Empowerment 75

TRUTH FOUR — 78
MONKEY SEE, MONKEY DO – ACTIONS SPEAK LOUDER THAN WORDS

- Mirror Neurons 78
- Empathy 80
- Developing Empathy in the Child.................................... 82
- Children as Spiritual Teachers 83
- Support the Parents of this World 85
- Parenting with Presence 86
- Self-control - A Predictor of Success 86

TRUTH FIVE — 91
OUR CHILDREN ARE CREATIVE FOUNTAINS

- The Creative Child... 91
- The Universe is our Playground 92
- Creativity... 93
- The Arts and Their Correlation With Scientific Brilliance 98
- Are Intelligence and Creativity Related? 99
- The Beauty of Boredom.. 102

TRUTH SIX *108*
UNCONDITIONAL LOVE IS A SUPERPOWER

- Defining Love 108
- Love is a Basic Human Need 110
- Our Children, the Canary in the Coal Mine 113
- It Takes a Village to Raise a Child 114
- Practicing Unconditional Love Towards Our Children ... 119
- The Pain of Shame 122
- Give the Child Space to Feel 124
- The Power of a Hug 125

TRUTH SEVEN *127*
YOU CAN'T POUR FROM AN EMPTY CUP

- Nurturing the Parent Carer or Role Model 127
- Change 129
- High Vibrational Emotions 135
- Divine Feminine 143
- Bathing our Children in Divinity 147

AFTERWORD *149*

ENDNOTES *153*

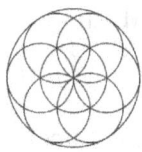

INTRODUCTION

'Children are the living messages we send to a time we will not see.'

John W. Whitehead
Human Rights Attorney

Raising children can be likened to an old man who plants an olive tree knowing that he may never reap the benefits of its fruit in his lifetime. Our children are the olive tree saplings that, through care and attention from their parents and elders, will grow into a stately tree from which abundant fruit will flourish. But it may be future generations, rather than the one who cared for this tree, who will enjoy its plentiful fruit.

For the plant to thrive it needs support stakes to grow straight and tall, abundant water and nourishment, and the presence of the sun's light and warmth. The tender seedlings are vulnerable and dependent, and without care will struggle to reach their full potential. We may not still be on this earthly plane to reap the full benefit of the care and effort that we invest in our own human seedlings, but knowing the benefits for humanity in the future should be reason enough to make this effort worth pursuing. This may be our only true opportunity to evoke meaningful, long lasting change.

Our children will take over the reins and steer humanity at a time in the not so distant future. Parenting, therefore, is one of the most crucial roles that we may perform. We are the artists, the children are our creative expression. The way we parent matters, and it is an opportunity to make one of the largest impacts on humanity that we may ever have.

For most of us, prior to having children, we were quite certain it couldn't possibly be that hard. Until you have kids, and you realise that:

1. I either have a moment of Divine intervention where everything is revealed to me in totality, or
2. I start reading a multitude of books.

Enter the books. When you start reading parenting books, you wish you'd had the spontaneous Divine intervention. The information is copious, and the recommendations on how to approach this gargantuan task often oscillate with societal shifts. I was intent on trying to find the 'answers' so that my children could hopefully one day uphold our decorated title of Homo sapiens...Latin for 'wise man'.

This journey of discovery started as a personal one, when I was attempting to demystify my new role as a parent. This is a responsibility held by so many of us, and I am yet to meet someone who has found it an easy journey. On this search for a unified approach to parenting I began to realise that there was a common thread that held together the complex tapestry of child-raising. Certain principles of parenting remain *eternally true*. The reason for writing this book was to compile these *eternal truths* that I wish I had known at the beginning of my journey into parenthood. These *eternal truths* form a magnificent golden thread that is woven into the tapestry of our parenting experience and the experience of our children.

There is a beauty and simplicity to this realisation. We have travelled full circle, and now science has provided the vernacular to explain the basis behind what we understood innately in a bygone time. The key to effective child-raising exists, and the elegance of this is that it has been tried and tested since the beginning of humankind.

Within the pages of this book you can explore the *eternal truths* of raising our adorable little primates. You can do this with the confidence that successful child nurturing is based on a handful of principles, that can be easily applied, and have been used repeatedly over time. I have stripped away the complexities to reveal fundamental principles that will provide a healthy bedrock for successful and fulfilling parenting.

What are eternal truths?

Eternal Truths are principles that are independent of rapid societal changes and are not based purely on opinion. These principles are firmly encoded within us as *biological expectations*. If we are able to uphold these simple truths, we are able to create a structurally sound foundation for our children, just as nature intended.

Determining what these *eternal truths* are has become important because societal changes are taking place with phenomenal rapidity. As the changes to society propel us forward, we find ourselves struggling to keep pace. This is mostly due to the fact that it is impossible for us to biologically adapt in the same time frame. On a societal and technological level we are powering ahead, but biologically we are the same as we were a couple of hundred thousand years ago.

When a baby Homo sapiens is born into this world, genetically he or she is programmed with the same expectations as a baby human born 300,000 years ago. Similarly the female body, soul and mind, all have certain needs that are part of a woman's biological expectations during the transformation from woman to mother. The same can be argued for fathers. It is therefore crucial to determine what these timeless biological expectations are, to ensure that they are fulfilled despite the fast pace we are traveling at collectively as a society.

The eternal truths of parenting promote qualities in ourselves and our children that sustain a meaningful and happy life. We are encoded with an innate wisdom of how to raise our young, but unfortunately this knowledge has been lost in the complexity of modern life. Once we peel away this convolution, and look at the essential components of raising well-adjusted, happy, content children, it becomes evident that parenting is not complicated after all, and we were designed to do it and to do it well.

We need to plan many generations ahead, and the way in which we raise our children is the planting of the seeds. The quality of our future is dependent on us developing integrated human beings. There is simplicity in the application of these principles, but the results are profound.

The 7 Eternal Truths

There are 7 Eternal Truths of Parenting, which cover the fundamentals of raising a Homo sapiens in the 21st century:

TRUTH 1:	Human babies and children have fundamental biological expectations
TRUTH 2:	What we inscribe in the child's mind will echo throughout their lifetime
TRUTH 3:	Parents are genetic engineers – epigenetics and engineering the future
TRUTH 4:	Monkey see, monkey do – actions speak louder than words
TRUTH 5:	Our children are creative fountains
TRUTH 6:	Unconditional love is a superpower
TRUTH 7:	You can't pour from an empty cup

In this book we will embark on a journey exploring each of these basic rules of bringing children into this world and raising them. We will uncover the eternal truths that we always knew, which become veiled behind the complexities of modern life. As we effectively remove the mist from the glass, we will see with clarity those aspects of raising children that are fundamental. These truths will become the foundational pillars upon which we can build a most rewarding and enjoyable parenting experience. It is time for us to relearn the basics of being a Homo sapiens, and relish the experience of raising these incredible creatures – our children.

Perfect parenting does not exist, and never will. Rather, it is a journey of the soul. We are thrust into the lives of each other, each as a Divine expression of what is right for that exact moment. Through the numerous obstacles that life presents, both the child and the parents begin their spiritual journey. Just as carbon turns into diamond under extreme pressure, so too are we given the opportunity to reach greatness through the experience of parenting.

A need to share and learn from each other

As our existence becomes increasingly nuclear, there arises a need for parents to share their experiences. Pregnancy, birth and child-raising were traditionally experienced in a communal setting, where support was common and the knowledge from the elders was easily accessible. This is rarely the case now; most parents are required to make important and far-reaching decisions in a state of semi-isolation.

By listening to the experiences of other women and men recounting their own journey through parenthood, we begin to reclaim the eternal truths. We will be able to observe patterns that will make our lives, and the lives of our children, easier. Everyone's personal account of his or her experience holds equal importance. This is because each experience, no matter how joyous or painful at the time, is an integral part of the complex interplay of the individual's own personal journey, as well as the journey of us all as a collective. *Everyone's* journey has purpose and meaning and can be a source of learning for others. Our experience of pregnancy, childbirth and parenting matters, and sharing and learning from those around you is an empowerment of the divine feminine - whether it is the experience of the mother or the father.

Family

Family structure does not fit within neat definitions, and need not do so. Our experience of family and what it can be is only enriched by the many beautiful variations of what constitutes a family unit. We all exist within a continuum of physical, emotional and spiritual expression. Each of us, whether we are male or female, embodies an expression of the divine feminine and divine masculine in varying degrees and this expression shifts for each individual over the duration of their life.

Various parts of this book at times focus on the role of the mother, since in the majority of situations the mother will be experiencing the pregnancy and birth of the child. This is not intended to isolate those who have non-biological children, or those who have not personally experienced the pregnancy or birth of their children. The application of the concepts of bonding and attachment flow into childhood, and the impact of this later time period cannot be emphasised enough.

The definition of *mother* beyond pregnancy and birth, is no longer confined to the one who conceived and birthed the child, but rather denotes the one who predominantly expresses the qualities of the divine feminine. A family unit, if woven with the essence of love, contains all that is needed to raise happy and contented children.

Why is parenting important?

The reason why the topics of conception, pregnancy, birth and early childhood are of such importance is because the ramifications of these experiences are not limited to those early years. Children are acutely sensitive to their experiences during each of these stages, the effects of which echo throughout their lifetime. In this way, we can begin to understand that through conscious and mindful child creation, we have the capacity to empower the whole of humanity.

We have seen the wonderful and much-needed expansion of information regarding methods of self-improvement, spirituality, and empowerment for adults. What if we were able to formulate a method of raising well-adjusted, confident, intelligent, conscious young children, as the next wave of humans who are to inherit this planet Earth? It could be argued that this is one of the most powerful capacities we have as parents and carers of our children.

The aim of the application of these principles is to amplify our life experience by creating loving bonds between the parent and child. This is the glue of humanity. Without it, society fragments. With it, the energy of a loving bond between the parent and child ultimately ripples throughout the whole of humanity. There is nothing of greater importance than parents ensuring they establish and maintain a loving bond with their children. And when we partake in this bond we realise that it is a source of incredible happiness, and it just feels beautiful. This, I maintain, is the natural state of parenting. And it is a state that we all have the innate capacity to experience.

A dance of the scientific and the spiritual

It becomes evident from the research, which we will explore in this book, that conscious parenting can be built on a strong framework of science. A conscious approach to the period from conception up to and including child-rearing no longer needs to be done on the premise of a 'gut feeling' alone. Through conscious parenting, we will witness the creation of children from whom love springs eternal.

The most fundamental platform upon which we have the capacity to create change is by virtue of our children. We now have science to describe many of the experiences of parenting. In addition, we are endowed with an innate, instinctual knowledge of how to raise our young. It is through this combination of science and instinct that we will be able to accelerate change in a positive direction.

How did we deviate from the eternal truths?

There are a few reasons why we have become disconnected from our inner wisdom regarding parenting. The main reason being the increasing complexity of our lives and the resulting disconnect from our inner selves. Additionally, there is an all-permeating culture of subtle denigration of roles that have been traditionally feminine. None of us are individually responsible for these societal shifts, but we are all affected by them. Once we acknowledge the root cause of the disconnect from our parental wisdom, we can make efforts to rejoin with it and reap the rewards.

As our society grows more complex, the need to create integrated human beings deepens. The information contained within this book is an exigency, as it is the most fundamental platform upon which we have the capacity to create change – by virtue of our children. It is through the symphony of a wholesome physical, mental and spiritual state in our children that we will see the true potential of humanity emerge in the future on a global scale.

Everyone will gain by raising peaceful, happy, thriving children. We have the power, through a conscious and informed approach to parenting, to change the trajectory of humanity – it is no less important than this. This will take place through an active desire on the part of parents who are aware of this urgency to rise above herd consciousness, to honour the role and accept the accountability of being the creators of our next generation.

My Wish For All Parents

By exploring the contents of this book I am hopeful that 'my wish for all parents' becomes a reality rather than a dream perceived as unattainable.

I wish that as parents, you will acknowledge your role in raising the next generation as one of the most profoundly influential things you can do.

I wish that parenthood will provide you with the challenges you need for your own mastery and that it provides you with an opportunity to learn more about your own true self.

I wish for you a firm realisation that although the child comes through you they are not of you.

I wish for you that you are able to practice wisdom, compassion and joy through the many forms that parenting takes.

I wish that on the path of parenting, you are able to connect with a deep wisdom, demonstrate compassion and experience a love of the greatest depth.

I wish that you can parent with clarity, and are guided by a deep knowing to distinguish between what is meaningless and what is meaningful.

I wish for you the ability to not lose sight of the forest for the trees, to continue to question the status quo and to live by your heart's calling.

I wish for you that the tapestry of your existence is woven with the strength to endure the painful and enjoy the ecstatic, with an understanding that each of the smaller melodies of experience make up the symphony of your parenting story.

I wish that you enjoy the simplest and quietest moments with your children as some of those with greatest depth, as you connect beyond the confines of your physical form.

I wish for you an understanding that will enable you to forgive and let go of the past, with the acceptance that life, no matter how messy, is a wonderful journey.

I wish for you the strength to live with love, and to release fear.

And I wish for you the belief that everything is unfolding exactly as it should, and that there is no need to pursue perfection, because everything *is* arising in complete perfection in the present moment.

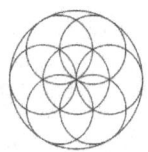

TRUTH ONE

The Human Foetus, Baby and Child have Fundamental Biological Expectations

Biological Expectations

It took 4.5 billion years for us to get to this moment, from the beginning of Earth's appearance. If the 4.5 billion years of Earth's existence were compressed into a 24-hour time line, humans emerged at 11.58pm. The entirety of human history has occurred within those last 2 minutes. This emphasises the brevity of our existence here on Earth, and the relatively short period in which we have experienced rapid change in the way we live.

It was only moments ago that our ancestors were hunter-gatherers, and now many of us live in nuclear families. This existence bears little resemblance to that of our earliest forebears. There are myriad reasons to be thankful for the comforts that many of us enjoy today, but we remain linked to our earliest origins by our DNA. An early Homo sapiens baby entered this world with certain expectations that would ensure their safe and healthy development into adulthood.

The *biological expectations* of a baby are more extensive than the mere survival *needs*. For survival, the *needs* are simple; clean water, nutrition, shelter, and basic human connection. Meeting *biological expectations* takes a step beyond merely meeting *needs*. It goes further by providing the framework for the child to thrive and develop their full innate human potential.

The biological expectations of babies have remained essentially unchanged for over three hundred thousand years. We must rediscover them and ensure that they are met within our modern circumstantial framework. This is an exciting endeavour in which we can be reminded of the essence of human existence. It is empowering to have the knowledge of what it is we *really* require, as parents and children, in order to fulfill our astounding potential.

What is our baby Homo sapiens expecting?

> *'Most mammals emerge from the womb like glazed earthenware emerging from a kiln – any attempt at remoulding will only scratch or break them. Humans emerge from the womb like molten glass from a furnace. They can be spun, stretched and shaped with a surprising degree of freedom. This is why today, we can educate our children to become Christian or Buddhist, capitalist or socialist, warlike or peace-loving.'*[1]
>
> Yuval Noah Harari
> *Sapiens - A Brief History of Humankind*

What distinguishes a baby Homo sapiens from other baby animals is that they are born more immature and helpless than any other living thing, and remain dependent for the longest period of time. Human babies are reliant on the adults closest to them for many years to ensure their survival and healthy development. In fact, it would be very difficult for a baby human to express their highest potential without these expectations being met.

Parents and carers of children are well aware of the intensity of raising them. If you didn't previously know that we birth the most dependent creature on the planet, you now have an explanation for the enormity of the responsibility! Once the baby arrives, there is no time to read, research and process the information on how to parent. After all, we are trying to keep this vulnerable little being content. Therefore, it becomes invaluable to understand what attention this child is expecting, and how we can fulfill those needs. By fulfilling the *biological expectations* of the child you are covering all their requirements to thrive, and there will be no further reason to ever doubt your parenting.

What are our children's fundamental biological expectations?

So what are these foundational requirements? Jean Leidloff, in her book *The Continuum Concept*[2], addresses the idea of a set of innate biological expectations that humans are genetically designed to experience during childhood. One could also argue that these biological expectations are also present during the time in utero and during the birthing process.

The most fundamental biological expectations of a child include:

- Being placed on the mother after birth, skin-to-skin
- Carrying and physical contact – in the first year the mother plays a very important role in this regard
- Being responded to when in need

- Sleeping in close proximity to the mother, ideally in a safe co-sleeping arrangement
- On-demand rather than scheduled feeding, ideally breastfeeding (where possible)

These expectations are inbuilt, strongly felt and, if not fulfilled, can endanger the healthy continuum that is necessary to build physically and psychologically sound adults. If these biological expectations are not met, it has been argued that one of the profound repercussions is that 'happiness ceases to be a normal condition of being alive, and becomes a goal.'[3]

Meeting biological expectations promotes attachment

Meeting Biological Expectations

⬇

Healthy Growth and Healthy Attachment (bonding)
Cultivating healthy body, mind and spirit in the child

A result of a child's biological expectations being met is the development of healthy attachment, also known as bonding, between the parent and child. The development of healthy attachment is a cornerstone of effective parenting. This topic is covered in detail later in this chapter. Once we compromise the basic biological expectations we blunt the means by which healthy attachment is created. Other than keeping the child alive, creating healthy attachment could be considered the whole aim of parenting. Without it, everything else crumbles.

At every stage in a child's development, it is profoundly important that we *maintain the steady progression of meaningful and loving bonding between the parent/carer and child*. This, I maintain, is the golden thread that binds each of the significant stages:

- Conception
- Pregnancy
- Childbirth
- Early childhood

The process of bonding in the early stages of child creation can have an effect on the future capacity of the child to love and accept love, including self-love. The ability to experience love is the single most important capability of any human being. Without the capacity to receive or express love, life becomes meaningless. We will discover in this chapter the forms that attachment takes, in each of the significant stages of parenting.

How have we deviated from what should arise instinctively?

The environment in which a baby Homo sapiens was born into 300,000 years ago, is significantly different to the environment into which a baby Homo sapiens is born into in the 21st century. However, the biological expectations with which the baby is born have remained eternal.

The exponential change that we have experienced post-industrialisation has resulted in our instinctive approach to raising children being at odds with societal expectations and obligations. In fact, the rate of change in our technologically dependent society has been so rapid that even the environment in which we grew up as children is significantly different to the one we experience as adults. The same will hold true for our own offspring, but to an even greater degree.

Despite this, it is heartening that it is possible to distil those elements of parenting that are most important. And by meeting those biological expectations and establishing healthy bonds with our children, we give ourselves the best chance of experiencing joyful parenting.

As more parents learn of the importance of applying this principle, we can restore its power, bringing it back into the collective psyche of our society. Through the recognition that raising well-adjusted children is of paramount importance to families and society as a whole, we will see its re-emergence as a priority within our culture.

We can ask ourselves, why does all this matter? Can't we just adopt changes to the way in which we experience pregnancy, birth and parenting to match the demands of our modern society? It is tempting and expedient to believe this is possible, but from a biological perspective this is not the case. We need to uncover and live the eternal truths that we know to be intuitively true, and in doing so meet the biological expectations of our children.

Attachment

'Bonding creates the sensory and emotional environment that shapes how we interpret and respond to relationships life long. Break the bond at the beginning and we set the stage for cycles of depression, anger, rage, substance abuse and violence, generation after generation.'[4]

James W. Prescott, Ph.D.
Brain and Behavioural Neuroscientist, Anthropologist

Attachment can be described as '...the enduring emotional bond between the child and parent, for which the stage is set from the moment the child is born...'[5] It is the formation of a connection dependent on closeness between two human beings. This is vital to many mammals and birds for survival of their offspring. It is of greatest importance to human infants as they are born the most helpless of any living thing on planet Earth. Attachment is paramount since it is vital for life. For a human baby, no attachment means no life.

We are programmed genetically to seek out those conditions that promote the development of attachment. A baby has a 'rooting reflex' where it seeks out the nipple of the mother after birth, and is soothed by the arms of a parent. A child regulates its breathing and heartbeat to that of the parent next to whom it sleeps. These behaviours enhance attachment, and this is not by coincidence. Babies and children are genetically coded to seek it out.

There are certain aspects of attachment that are vital for us to understand, in order to optimise our bonding experiences with our children. I explain each in the following pages.

You cannot over-attach

You cannot love your child too much. The process of attachment does not create children who are more needy or insecure. The way to create children who eventually display independence and maturity is to initially provide the means for attachment. As Gordon Neufeld, Ph.D and Gabor Mate, M.D. in their book 'Hold On to Your Kids' state: '...the story of maturation is one of paradox: *dependence and attachment foster independence and genuine separation.*'[6]

Invest time in attaching and bonding with your baby and child, as it will result in healthy independence. This is not a process that happens quickly, and could extend beyond the teenage years.[7]

We need to rise above the common misconception that the earlier the child displays independence the better. There is a time for every stage, and there is no need to desire that the child develop maturity and independence beyond his or her years.

Attachment is the foundation for healthy psychological development

Babies and children look to us as emotional barometers. We are vital for the development of their ability to navigate within society. These skills cannot be learnt from peers, and are dependent upon the knowledge and wisdom of the parents, carers and other influential adult figures.

It is essential that the child builds a sense of security by knowing their human compass is there to support them in learning how to move through this world. Without access to this, the child is adrift and at the mercy of the direction and role modelling provided by other ill-equipped children or the nearest adult figure to whom they can attach.[8]

You need to be present to attach to the child

We are facing a unique point in human history where children spend a very high percentage of their waking day in the presence of other children, and many adults who are not from the family unit. This situation emerged after the industrial revolution. How it arose is the subject of a complex societal discussion, but we have all found ourselves within a system that champions the separation of children from their family during the majority of the working week to enable the parents to partake in the paid workforce.

It may be obvious to state this fact, but you must be physically present with your child in order for attachment to take place. It is a simple truth. It is necessary for society to offer support to parents who need to spend time attaching with their children. Particularly with school age children, parents must recognise the need to spend time after school to reestablish attachment with the child.

If you are not attaching with your child, the child will fill the void with someone or something else

All children need to attach to someone. They are biologically hardwired to attach. If you are not present to bond with your child, the child either attaches to other suitable adult figures in their vicinity, such as teachers, or in unfortunate situations, to other children as their role models. It is vital for you to ask yourself, 'Who is my child attaching to and how well do I know them?' because when you are not present, they are attaching to someone else.

Healthy attachment to parents or carers is vital for the development of well-adjusted, secure children who will, at the right time, exhibit healthy and confident independence. It can be argued that this is the most important role of the parent, since without this vital psychological development of the child, ultimately the whole fabric of society is threatened.

Other children are obviously unsuitable attachment figures, but we can safely say that there is currently a strong culture of peer attachment, particularly amongst teens. This peer attachment is replacing the social structure that has been the backbone of the survival of humankind. What is most important for the healthy development of the child is the formation of attachment to suitable adult figures. Without this the child will not have any desire to follow the direction or advice of the parent or carer; rather, they will follow the direction and advice of the peer group.

It is a common complaint of many parents with teenage children that they feel a lack of connection with the child. With this loss of connection between parents and children, we begin to witness a loss of social structure and culture. The result is many children who are adrift, or who become disciples of their peer groups, with the older generations becoming irrelevant in their worldview. Since this is the predominant nature of peer group relationships in our current western culture, it is widely accepted as normal. Unfortunately this is neither normal nor healthy. Rather, it is a social adaptation to our contemporary cultural trends. These trends are at odds with the formation of healthy attachment relationships between children and their parents or older role models.

Most children will undertake their education in a system in which they are grouped together with peers, with a very low teacher to child ratio. The odds of peer attachment are very high in this scenario. We must then ask ourselves what we can do as well-intending parents to nurture the attachment and bonding with our children. The answer is that we need to commit time and effort to *re-attaching* with our child after each period of separation. This takes commitment and habit. Another approach is to ensure weekends are devoted to re-attachment with your children rather than participating in strings of peer-oriented activities. It is worth every effort to re-enforce the attachment between parent and child.[9]

Quantity over quality

Integral to all of this is being present with the child. And (although it may seem counter-intuitive) it is usually quantity that matters more than quality. All the child needs is your presence; from that will stem the beautiful process of bonding. Without sufficient time, there is limited opportunity for bonding to unfold. Unfortunately, for many parents, time is a limited commodity. But in parenting, time is what matters above all else. Without a time-commitment to the early years of parenting, you run the risk of a lifetime of remedial parenting once the child has disconnected.

By honouring the process of attaching with your child you will deepen your bonding, and this can be argued as being the most rewarding experience of a parent, because it is a gift that keeps giving over an entire lifetime.

Attachment at Different Stages of the Parenting Journey

It is important to look at the various stages of child raising, to determine what form attachment and bonding takes at these different points, and how it affects the development of the infant or child. There are things we can do at each of these stages to promote wholesome attachment. I will now discuss the pivotal processes that take place at major turning points of child creation – namely conception, pregnancy, birth and childhood, and explain how each stage affects bonding between parent and child.

Conception and Pregnancy

> *'Awake or asleep, the studies show, [unborn children] are constantly tuned in to their mother's every action, thought and feeling. From the moment of conception, the experience in the womb shapes the brain and lays the groundwork for personality, emotional temperament, and the power of higher thought.'*[10]
>
> Dr Thomas R. Verny, M.D.
> **Founder of the Association for Prenatal and Perinatal Psychology and Health**

Bonding with your child starts from the time of conception; some may believe, even prior to this. The architecture of the brain is developed during the time in utero and beyond. As we are aware, bonding is the creation of a close, long-lasting relationship between two people as a result of frequent or continuous association. No other relationship is closer or more frequent than the relationship between the mother and her unborn child.

Women have the capacity to change the trajectory of humanity, and this is an innate power that all pregnant women need to become aware of. Building this relationship with the baby in utero, or even prior to conception, is not a foreign concept in many traditional cultures. An example of this is the Native American belief of building a notion in your mind of what you wish your child to be:

'To her poetic mind the imminent birth of her child prefigures the advent of a great spirit – a hero, or the mother of heroes – a thought conceived in the virgin breast of primeval nature, and dreamed out in a hush broken only by the sighing of the pine tree of the thrilling or orchestra of a distant waterfall.'[11]

Ohiyesa
Santee Dakota Physician, Writer, National Lecturer and Reformer

We need to genuinely ask ourselves what future we wish to create for this world and then consciously provide the environment for the child in utero to reach that potential.

The mother's emotions bathe the unborn child

'...incoming signals - crystallized through the mother as a swirl of behaviour, sensation, feeling, and thought - immerse the unborn child in a primordial world of experience, continuously directing the development of the mind.'[12]

The previously adopted view of the child's mind being a *tabula rasa* or 'blank slate' at the time of birth is erroneous. We are well aware that at the time of birth, the baby's brain contains approximately 100 billion neurons[13] (as many stars as there are in the Milky Way), and that many intricate neuronal connections are developed during pregnancy.

Environmental influences such as nutrients (the foods we consume), disease-causing microorganisms and toxins can all have an effect on foetal development. Another area of influence that cannot be ignored is the impact of the mother's emotional state on the development of the unborn child. The architecture of the brain is determined by an interplay between genetics and experience, including our experience in utero. The result of this interplay between environmental impacts and the mother's emotional state 'fires and wires' a certain set of neuronal connections within the brain of the foetus. It will be this neuronal network that acts as the bedrock for *all* future experiences.

The feelings and emotions of the mother are translated into hormonal and chemical signals which career through the blood stream. These signals eventually pass across the placenta into the bloodstream of the foetus. Hormones, neurotransmitters and polypeptides flow throughout the foetal brain and are one way in which the pregnant mother communicates with the child.[14] As adults 'these same molecules...determine whether we are prone to depression, joy, anxiety or calm.'[15] The consequences of being primed for certain emotional states in utero can be explained thus:

A predisposition for certain emotions (in response to triggers) impacts behavioural patterns. These patterns can be described as our personality. And our personality determines how we experience life in general.

Stress is an emotion where either physical, emotional or psychological change causes strain. The main hormones involved in the stress response are glucocorticoids and catecholamines. In the short-term, these hormones are protective, but in the case of long-term, chronic release, they can be damaging. Research is now showing that increased emotional stress during pregnancy may lead to dysregulation of the stress response system.[i]

The negative effects of a disrupted stress response system on the foetus have been studied in both animals and humans and include increased risk for compromised neurodevelopment, long term emotional, behavioural and psychiatric disorders[16] and poor birth outcomes.[17]

If the hormones of stress are present in excessive amounts at sensitive periods of the foetus' development, the brain and body of the foetus will act hyper-responsively to stress signals, and this will continue post birth and into adulthood. On the contrary, a foetus that is receiving primarily molecules that are the language of love, joy and calmness, will be primed to predominantly feel and exhibit those emotions, in utero and beyond.[18]

The foetus' brain is in a period of incredibly rapid development in utero. There are 50,000 neurons being formed every second in the baby in utero. During this period the brain is very vulnerable to stressors and these delicate connections can be easily destroyed.[19] It is the production of cortisol by the mother, when in a state of stress, which can be destructive to these delicate neurons. This limits the capacity of these neurons to fulfill their complete genetic potential. The quality

---

i   The two main stress response systems are the Hypothalamic–Pituitary–Adrenal (HPA) Axis and the Autonomic Nervous System (ANS).

and development of the infant's brain is heavily influenced by the mother's emotional state.

The period of conception and pregnancy are fundamentally important in the process of hard-wiring the child's brain. The foetal brain is 'fired and wired' together in preparation for the type of world the mother perceives she is experiencing. In this way the mother's role is as powerful as being the mother of the whole of humanity, since through her prevailing influence, we are the architects of our future. The outside world is impressing on the child's brain from the moment of conception, via the molecules of emotion of the mother. If we want a peaceful future for humanity, the child needs hormonal and chemical signals from the mother indicating that the external environment is one of peace.

In many traditional cultures, the period of pregnancy was regarded as a hallowed time. This is in stark contrast to the practices of modern western society. Over time we have distanced ourselves from connecting to our inner wisdom or our intuition. We need to return to our innate understanding that conception and pregnancy matter profoundly, and mothers need the affection, love and support necessary to create a peaceful and loving humanity.

Conscious conception and pregnancy

> *'Woman is the artist of the imagination and the child in the womb is the canvas whereon she painteth her pictures.'*
>
> Paracelsus (1493-1541)
> **Swiss Physician, Alchemist, Lay Theologian and Philosopher of the German Renaissance**

The concept of experiencing a 'conscious' conception and pregnancy is a spiritual description of being mentally in a place of *awareness* or *presence* in the existing moment. It is also being in a state of *mindfulness* of one's choices during this time, and being observant of one's thoughts and emotions.

It is not a new concept to nurture a pregnant woman, and to understand that she needs the time and space for optimum nutrition and calmness. These practices have been upheld traditionally for many thousands of years in many cultures. Unfortunately in the modern western world, we are finding that many women are sacrificing the celebration of the innate feminine and sacredness of human creation during pregnancy.

Women are not necessarily the perpetrators of these choices, but rather the victims of a society that is failing to recognise the importance of this role and therefore not providing adequate support to those who wish to focus on this time as one of paramount importance. I have myself been a pregnant woman, working night shifts in an emergency department. No one acknowledged the pregnancy, I worked as though I was not pregnant, and there is often no option for a woman to take time to focus on the sacred work she is doing. What I have since learnt is that pregnancy is a superpower. And any woman undergoing this process of creation should be venerated as such. It is miraculous.

It is time that the work of the feminine in human creation is once again acknowledged, revered and upheld as one of the most important things that she can do – this I believe, is true feminism. It is not denying the feminine, but embracing, maintaining and giving it the respect it deserves. Through this adoration of the feminine, we provide mothers with the support necessary to begin the process of bonding and attachment with their unborn child.

Birth – Bringing Human Consciousness into this World

'If a woman doesn't look like a Goddess during labor, then someone isn't treating her right.'

Ina May Gaskin
Midwife, Author

Birth is a sacred process by which we bring human consciousness into this world. It is the culmination of one of the most miraculous examples of creation. And with each birth we witness a spark of hope for humanity. Birth is a sensitive time where the bonding process between mother and baby should occur without interruption as far as possible. All births are sacrosanct, and whether the birth is a vaginal delivery or a caesarean, there are various methods to ensure that effective bonding is established between mother and child.

Birth provides us with a flowering of a multitude of moments of creating attachment between the mother and baby. After all, both the mother and the baby are awash in the hormones of love and bonding. This creates a foundation upon which a rich and fulfilling attachment between the baby and the parents can be built.

It is always important to keep in mind that there are many factors that come into play during the process of birth. We are complex beings and no woman should ever be judged for her birth choices. Life can take twists and turns seemingly completely out of our control at times, and many factors can influence our birth choices and the way in which birth unfolds. There are also women who don't experience the births they had wished for. This is not a failure. Every single woman's birthing experience is an important expression of the divine feminine, no matter what form it takes or what choices she makes. A woman giving birth is undergoing the sacred process of creating another life form, and any woman who undertakes this should be honoured.

Every woman's voice counts. Every woman's birth story marks a moment of individual transformation and is something that we can gain insight from. It is important that women continue to be heard, and that they can express their birthing experiences free of judgment, as *every* woman's birth story is significant and important. It is imperative that women listen to each other's experiences with an open mind and heart, as doing this empowers and strengthens the divine feminine.

For many of us who have had more than one child, we understand that no two births are the same. I am forever grateful to all the women who took the courage to share their very personal birth stories, whatever form it had taken, as it was from their experiences that I was able to find strength and courage to meet the demands of bringing new life into this world.

Childbirth and bonding

Mother-infant bonding is common to all mammals and involves interplay of various behaviours between the mother and baby. As we are well aware, the formation and maintenance of healthy bonding between humans is the foundation for a healthy society. For this reason the discussion of the seminal moment of bond formation between the mother and child at birth is critical.

It has been suggested that the quality of bonding between mother and child in the initial moments after birth has far-reaching and long-lasting effects on the life of the baby and mother. Michel Odent, a well-known French obstetrician and natural birth advocate, has proposed that there is a link between the capacity to love *oneself* and the ability to love *others*. Odent emphasises the sensitive period after birth as having a strong influence on one's ability to love oneself and love others later in life.[20]

The capacity to love oneself, accept love from those around you, and, in turn, show love, could possibly be the foundation of our life experience. A life with a diminished capacity to love is a life not experienced at its fullest magnitude.

We can begin to comprehend the ripple effect throughout our lifetime of effective bonding, and how crucial this is. Not only is our own life experience dependent on it, but also due to our interconnection with all people and things surrounding us, our Earth is dependent on it. Adequate early bonding provides an opportunity for the human brain to be optimally primed with the ability to love. These bonds of affection will expand love and the effect of this will ripple out and raise the vibrations of humanity. It is no less important than this.

The delicate hormonal interplay during labour and birth

To understand the process of bonding and attachment at birth, it is useful to have an appreciation of the birthing hormones. There is great complexity of the hormonal interplay during labour and birth. The picture is not entirely complete and there is still more to be learnt about the intricacies of this process. What is evident though, is that this balance is very delicate, and a respect for the natural unfoldment of birthing, where possible, can result in positive outcomes for the mother and child.

There are a few hormones that require special mention as they are integral to the process of birth and the bonding that occurs between the mother and baby after birth. I will explore their main features below.

Oxytocin

Oxytocin, the love hormone, is the major hormone in birth that stimulates uterine contractions. Oxytocin is not only limited to birthing, but is also secreted during breastfeeding, love making and male and female orgasm. It is also linked to sensitive caregiving.[21] Oxytocin is the master hormone in the role of bond formation.[22] The importance of this hormone has been broadened recently with suggestions that it underpins the biochemical basis of sociability and is responsible for social cohesion.[23]

Oxytocin is produced in the hypothalamus, and is released into the systemic circulation via the posterior region of the pituitary gland located in the brain. During the birthing process, there is a positive feedback loop in which the oxytocin produces contractions of the uterus. Oxytocin is also responsible for the milk let down reflex of the lactating mother.

Beta-endorphin

Beta-endorphin, a naturally occurring opiate, affects the way in which women experience pain during labour. High levels of this hormone are present during pregnancy, birth and breastfeeding. When we experience stress, this hormone is released and can result in feelings of pleasure, euphoria and ecstasy. You can witness the high levels of beta-endorphin reached in a woman during a natural birth as an altered state of consciousness. It is as though the birthing mother is in another world – and this is typically seen in an undisturbed birth.

As pain increases in birth, so do the levels of beta-endorphin and this then inhibits oxytocin release, slowing contractions. It is an inbuilt mechanism to ensure that the intensity of the contractions does not exceed the level that the woman can cope with. In addition to helping the woman cope with labour, beta-endorphin plays an integral role in the initial relationship between the mother and baby and in initiating breastfeeding.[24]

Adrenaline and Noradrenaline (Catecholamines)

These are the 'fight-or-flight' hormones' that are released from the adrenal glands, small triangular glands located on top of each kidney. These hormones are released in response to stressful events. The interesting thing about these catecholamines is that they have a different effect at various points in the labour process. In the initial stages it has the effect of inhibiting oxytocin, thereby slowing down progression.

During labour it is crucial to create an environment that is not stressful for the woman. This would have been an essential mechanism in the past, when women birthed in an environment that had the risk of predators. In such a situation it would have been imperative for the labour to slow or stop to ensure survival of the mother and baby. In the later stage of labour when birth is about to take place, a surge in catecholamines is vital for the final ejection of the baby.

Prolactin

This hormone is the 'mothering' hormone, and peaks at the time of birth. Prolactin is the main hormone for breast milk production. It is also responsible for creating the emotion of putting the baby's needs first. Prolactin and oxytocin, are powerful hormones for the initial bonding between the mother and baby.

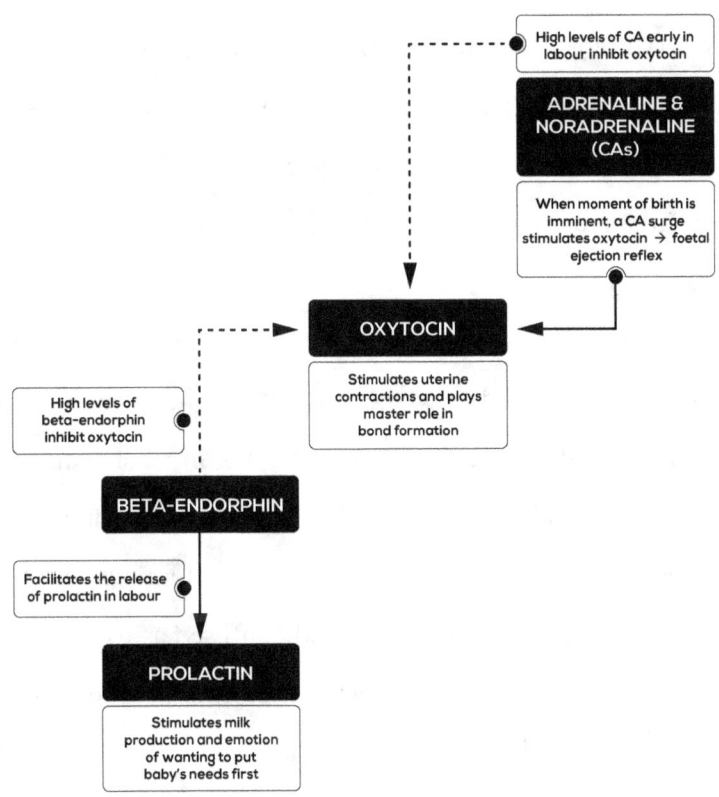

Diagram 1: Overview of the interrelationship of the main hormones of birth.
Note: Dotted arrows represent inhibition and solid arrows represent stimulation.

The effects of interfering with the labour process

There is a fine interplay between the various hormones of birth, each with a specific and pivotal role in ensuring the well-being of the mother and baby. There are various obstetric interventions that can disrupt this exquisite hormonal orchestra. It also becomes evident that once birth is interfered with, we often witness a succession of events each needing further intervention. It then becomes easy to get carried along on the torrent of medical intervention – and many women become another statistic in the high rates of caesarean sections, which continue to trend upwards. We then have the unfortunate situation of many well-intending mothers finding themselves in a situation of experiencing less than optimal bonding with their baby.

On the following page in Table 1, I have outlined the most common obstetric interventions and how they can affect the process of bonding with the mother. There is a cost to disrupting the innate hormonal flow in a labouring woman, and this cost could be higher than we initially thought.

Many women enter the hospital with the best intentions for themselves and their baby, but leave overwhelmed and confused as to what has taken place. Not only that, they are left to their own devices, to process a birth that has unfolded with very little support and not according to plan. Postnatal depression affects up to 1 in 7 women in the first year after birth and anxiety is likely to be at least as common.[25]

Although the causes of postnatal depression are complex, it has been shown in studies that among women with no history of depression, undergoing instrument-assisted or caesarean delivery, there is increased risk.[26] This is a very important consideration since postnatal depression can result in negative personal and child development outcomes.[27]

OBSTETRIC PROCEDURE	WHAT IT IS USED FOR	HOW IT CAN INTERFERE WITH BONDING
Synthetic Oxytocin	Induction of labour, Speed up labour	Can interfere with the natural oxytocin levels in mother and child.[28],[29] Decreases effectual breastfeeding by inhibiting several associated primitive neonatal reflexes.[30]
Opioids (Morphine/Pethidine)	Pain relief – it is still used even though it provides limited pain relief.[31]	Has been shown to reduce the woman's own opioid production and can directly reduce the release of oxytocin.[32] Can impair early breastfeeding (due to sedating effects on the infant)[33]
Epidural Analgesia	Pain relief	Reduces natural oxytocin.[34] Can affect breastfeeding by disturbing baby's suckling reflexes.[35]
Caesarean	Surgical intervention	Maternal peaks of oxytocin, endorphins, catecholamines and prolactin are lowered or absent. Breastfeeding often delayed.[36] Effects of mother's post-operative pain relief on baby through breastmilk.

Table 1: Overview of the effect of obstetric intervention on optimal bonding between the mother and baby post birth.

In her book *Gentle Birth, Gentle Mothering,* Dr Sarah Buckley[37] comprehensively details the negative effect of the various forms of intervention, with the research regarding each. I would highly recommend this book if you are interested in the details of the effects of various forms of obstetric intervention.

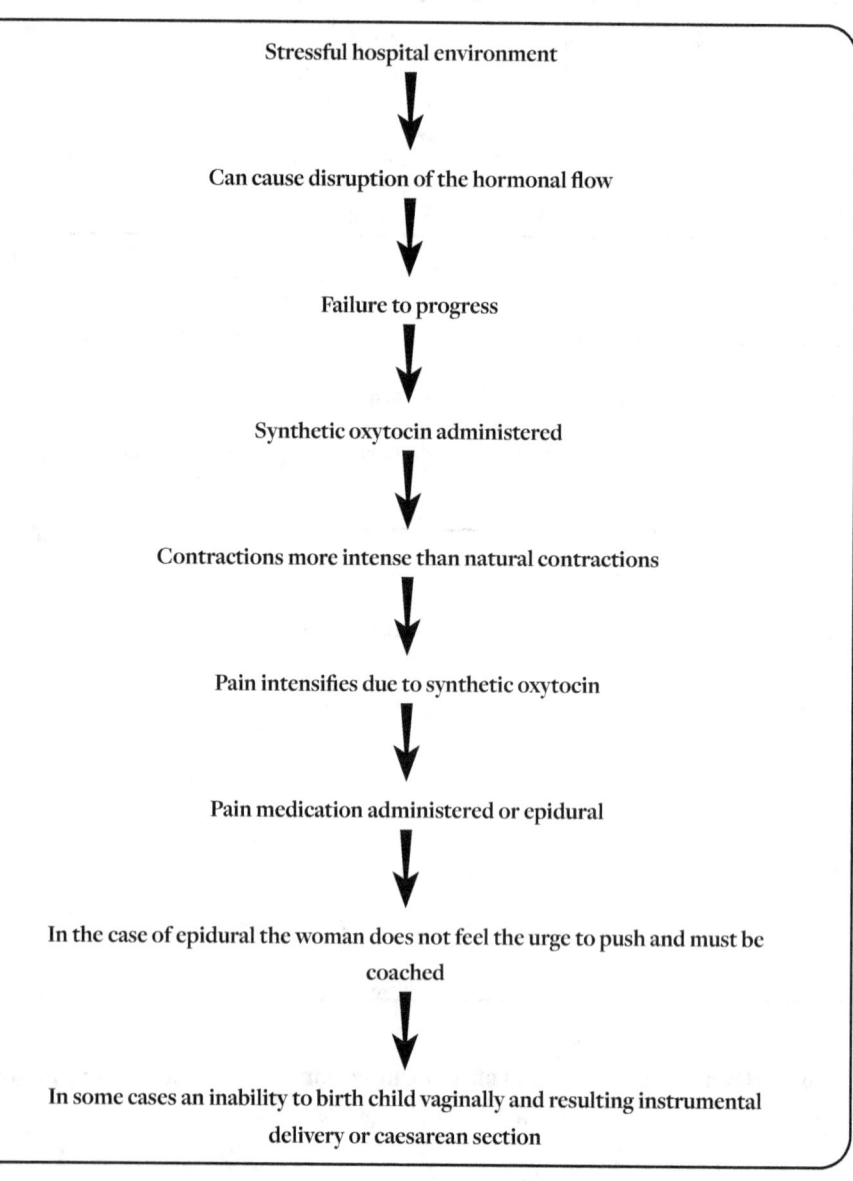

Diagram 2: Possible domino effect of a medicalised birth

Birthing choices

There are instances where births require particular interventions for the safety and well-being of the mother and child. Modern medicine has been a saviour in providing the means and knowledge for interventionist care when required. There are various reasons why a caesarean birth is the most ideal option for some women. This can include:

- Certain medical conditions
- Previous trauma - whether that be a previous birth or other trauma (such as sexual violence)
- The mother feels this is the best option for her and her baby

There are a multitude of reasons a person's birth experience takes a particular form, and every birth is sacred. There are ways to ensure optimal attachment between mother and child at the time of birth no matter what form the birth takes.

Gentle caesarean

There are now options to experience a 'gentle caesarean' or 'natural caesarean.' Here, certain changes are made to the surgical environment to emphasise the patient-centred approach to birthing. This is a wonderful option for women who would like to experience the process of early attachment with the baby, as early as possible after the birth. This would be a discussion worth having with your health care provider if a caesarean is planned. With collaboration between the various members of the team during the cesarean, a gentle caesarean is possible.[38]

A gentle caesarean can involve changes to the environment in the operating theatre such as:[39]

- Dimming the lights
- Warming the room
- Providing the infant with a warming blanket post birth
- Gentle music

Visiting the theatre prior to the procedure can be helpful. In addition, you can organise:

- The presence of more than one support person
- A person of choice to cut the umbilical cord
- Immediate and continued skin-to skin contact post birth[40]
- Encouragement of breastfeeding in the operating theatre[41]

These are wonderful options to promote early bonding and attachment between mother and baby in those acute and sensitive moments right after birth.

Natural vaginal birth

If a mother has experienced a healthy and full term pregnancy, natural birth is an option. Many would argue that medical assistance is preferable to the experience of the pain and uncertainty of a natural birth; however, uninterrupted birthing optimises effective bonding and attachment between the mother and baby. It is within these bonds of affection that love will flourish.

For those who feel that natural birth is an option that suits their health and psychological situation, I explore below the ways in which an expectant mother and her support group can optimise her chances of experiencing a natural birth.

Pain and childbirth

Let's start with the aspect of pain in childbirth. This is usually the first thing that springs to mind when we think about birth. Our conditioning by popular media has ensured that we view birth with fear and trepidation. The decision to opt for a natural birth is sometimes a difficult discussion since we are naturally inclined to pursue situations that are comfortable and predictable. In childbirth, pain is baulked at, yet it is championed in other aspects of our society's endeavours - a perfect example being extreme pursuits in sport. We need to develop a dialogue that respects the pain in childbirth as an expression of an extension of our usual capabilities.

Pain of childbirth as functional

From a purely physiological perspective, the pain of childbirth is functional. As we discover more about the delicate interplay of the hormones of birth, we can see how the sensation of pain is involved. Oxytocin is the hormonal driver of the birthing process. As the levels of oxytocin increases, the contractions of the muscular uterus increase in frequency and intensity. This is what causes the sensation of pain during labour. This *pain with a purpose* is a result of things going *right*, not of things going *wrong*. This is in contrast to pathological pain, where it is an indication that something is wrong. It is important for women to understand this distinction.

Once the levels of pain reach a peak point, it is a signal to the body to release endorphins. These are our natural opiates. This moderates the pain and the woman shifts from her conscious/thinking mind to her deeper/instinctual mind, in which she is able to reach to her greatest depths to experience the birth. Moving into this mind takes her to a raw, primal space. This is an experience in which you can reach for an innate power; one which you may never have known resided within you. It is here that dwells a tremendous strength. It is as though, in this space, we are re-enacting the birth of the universe – the ultimate creative act of giving new life.

It is *pain* that is necessary to get us to that point. If we interfere with the process of pain during birthing, we can impede the unfolding of this intricate interplay of the physiology of birth, and effectively deny ourselves what can be a most empowering experience.

The experience of birth in a patriarchal medical system

It is true that most women now experience the process of birth within a system built on the foundations of patriarchy, the attitudes and practices of which still echo through hospitals today. It is a system that would have viewed the raw, primal nature of birthing as inconvenient, and confronting. As many women birth in a hospital that is designed to deal with pathology, it is not surprising that the pain of childbirth has become confused with the pain of pathological conditions.

This distinction is fundamental – the pain of childbirth is normal, functional pain whereas the pain of pathological conditions is a different beast altogether. We must remind ourselves that childbirth, in its natural and healthy state, is on the normal spectrum of human physical suffering.

Birth in its natural state is raw, primal and powerful. These are not images that sit neatly within the medical system. Birth is uncomfortable, unpredictable in nature, and requires patience and observation of the process. These are all characteristics that don't sit harmoniously within a medical system which likes to maintain tight control. Rather than allowing women to experience their physical peak and innate power, we have a medical culture that muffles the experience of bringing new life to Earth. We not only dull the woman's experience of birthing, but we also dull the baby's experience of birth, as we know the drugs used in medicalised births also career through the bloodstream of the baby.

It is undeniable that the medical system is indispensable in cases of a pathological birth - a birth that does not sit comfortably within the spectrum of a normal, healthy birth - but it is also undeniable that we are medicalising a process that for many women is not pathological. In doing so, it is imperative that we question what is lost for those women, who then endure the impacts of needless interference with the birthing process.

Pain and suffering as a transformative experience

It is the case that some women do not experience pain as such during childbirth, and some are lucky enough to experience what has been described as an 'orgasmic birth', but here I can only speak from my own experience. Reflecting upon the births of my daughters, I was filled with total fascination that birthing was such a life-changing experience, yet an experience common to so many women throughout time.

For the first time in my life, I had experienced a pain so intense that the only way to go through it was to surrender to it completely. Herein lay the transformation through the pain of birth – it was almost a microcosmic spiritual awakening. I had to yield in my entirety and have faith in the human design. It was reclamation of a power that I did not know existed within me. And once discovered, it is a power that is never lost. It is one manifestation of the divine feminine power.

Every woman should be allowed the opportunity to make the choice to experience a birth undisturbed, and be given the support, space and time for this to take place – if she so wishes. The pain of childbirth should be allowed to exist as acceptable within the normal spectrum of human suffering, if the birthing mother so chooses.

Creating a birth-friendly environment

If you wish to experience a birth undisturbed, there are a number of things you can do to the environment that will support this process. There is a complex and delicate interplay between the hormones of birth. For birth to proceed naturally it is vital that the right amount of birth hormones are produced at the appropriate times during the birthing process. Understanding the areas of the brain involved in the birth process allows us to appreciate the aspects of the brain we need to utilise and that which we need to quieten to birth naturally. I will discuss two areas of the brain, the limbic system and the neocortex and how they are involved in our experience of birth.

Limbic system

The limbic system, also called the middle or mammalian brain, is involved in our emotional and behavioural responses and is unique to mammals. This part of the brain is mainly involved in the behaviours that are necessary for survival such as the fight or flight response, reproduction, caring for our young, and feeding. The hippocampus and amygdala are the two main parts of the limbic system. Oxytocin, beta-endorphin, the catecholamines and prolactin are primarily produced by the limbic system within the brain.

Neocortex

The neocortex is involved in higher mental functions such as sensory perception, cognition, memory, language, generation of motor commands and conscious thought. The neocortex is a structure with tremendous information-processing and information-storing capacity. All aspects that differentiate us from other animals are contained within this region of the brain.. It is the neocortex that is the source of rational thought, empathy, love, compassion and altruism.[42]

Preparing for a natural birth by quieting the neocortex

The release of the four major hormones of birthing – oxytocin, beta-endorphin, catecholamines and prolactin are regulated by the limbic system. For birth to proceed naturally it is essential that the woman's energy is less focused on the rational, thinking neocortex brain, and allows the limbic system to work its magic. This can be a challenging thing to do when many of us are used to being 'in control', and feel uneasy if we are not.

Michel Odent spoke of their practice at Pithivers, a French hospital, which emphasised the importance of this: 'On the day of birth we encourage women in labor to give in to the experience, to lose control, to forget all they have learned – all the cultural images, all the behavioral patterns.'[43] In fact quieting the neocortex could be the cornerstone of achieving a natural birth.

We find that in a typical hospital setting, the neocortex is being stimulated, which effectively draws the birthing woman back into her thinking brain (the neocortex), which can slow the progression of labour.

If an animal is interrupted during the birthing process it can interfere with the progression of the labour. Humans are no different. The environment in which a woman is giving birth should be one in which she would feel safe making love. This should be the standard applied to determine if the birthing environment is conducive to an optimized birthing experience. The environment is pivotal in quieting the mind and subduing the preconceptions and fear that many women carry with them about birth.

Birth has become so heavily medicalised and is viewed as a process to be feared. It is important that women work through, and overcome, these beliefs prior to the birthing process. Women need to be in a relaxed and calm state of surrender, free from fear and doubts.

There are a number of things that can be done to achieve a sense of privacy and safety for the mother. This will encourage an effective mix of the birthing hormones to be released, in turn promoting a gentle birth.

- The environment should ideally be one that encourages a sense of safety and familiarity. This is more difficult to achieve in a hospital setting, but is easily achieved in a homebirth. Birthing centres, if available, provide a suitable middle ground for those not comfortable with a homebirth.
- Keep the lighting low – by keeping the room dimly lit we are creating a private environment that will be minimally stimulating to the neocortex.

- Talking to or communicating with a labouring woman should be kept to a bare minimum. By talking to a labouring woman, you are effectively pulling her out of the state of 'going within' and stimulating the neocortex. If you observe a woman in natural advanced labour, she appears as though she is in another world. A woman should not be interrupted during this period of deep surrender. This is representative of a reduction in the neocortical activity.
- Keep ambient noise and other auditory stimulation to a minimum. This is important to consider in a hospital setting where there are various pieces of equipment that may be at work.
- Avoid excessive examinations of the labouring woman. Again this will stimulate neocortical activity and can result in the release of adrenaline, which can slow labour.
- Make sure the labouring woman doesn't feel 'observed'. This again stimulates the neocortex and can therefore slow the progression.

It is essential that the right combination of birthing hormones are released at the right time in the right amounts, and this delicate balance is strongly influenced by the environment in which the woman is placed. For any woman wishing to experience an undisturbed birth, dedication to creating an environment of minimal stimulation and distraction is of paramount importance.

Love your body's ability to birth

It is impossible to deny the innate feminine power when witnessing a woman giving birth to new life. No matter what form the birth takes, it is time for women to regain confidence in the birthing process, support each other in this expression of the divine feminine, and to do what is necessary to promote attachment with this new human being. Birth should be approached as being a wonderful and safe experience and during birth, we must have the innate knowing that with the passing of each moment the baby is being brought closer and closer to you.

The First Moments After Birth

This precious time is one of wonder, awe and love. These delicate first hours post birth are crucial since the baby and mother are awash in hormones that precipitate healthy bonding for years to come.[44] The importance of attachment has been researched over the years and it has been found that in animals and juvenile delinquents 'intense mother-child attachment was a requirement for psychological wholeness. Without it...disorders of the brain and psyche would result.'[45] The importance of this process cannot be overstated. It is in the best interests of the mother, baby and society that this time is honoured and that all is done in our power to create the best possible environment for bonding between the mother and baby.

The first hour after the birth is a particularly sensitive time for the bonding and attachment process between mother and baby.[46] During this time, the mother and baby's systems, although now physically separate, are still awash in the hormones of birth, particularly endorphins, which play an important role in the attachment process.

The main hormone responsible for the initiation of postnatal bonding is oxytocin. This is not only involved with the process of breastfeeding, but as more oxytocin is released, the love between the mother and baby grows. It is called the hormone of love for this reason. By providing the baby with love, a sense of safety and reassurance, combined with the powerful effects of oxytocin, you are setting up the perfect environment for bonding to occur. The effects of this are long-lasting.

If we prioritise the importance of creating healthy bonds between the mother and child, it will undoubtedly affect society as a whole, since the way the child will interact with the world later in life will be influenced by the way they experience love and relationships during their early years. If a baby is given optimal bonding as a child, it will encourage the development of the ability to love freely and to receive love as an adult. What more could one ask for in this lifetime? The neuropsychological implications of effective bonding cannot be overemphasised.

Touch

Skin-to-skin contact is a most beautiful and love-inducing sensation between mother and child. Post birth, the baby's nervous system is primed to receive this wondrous feeling. The skin is the largest organ of our body. When skin is touched, the pressure receptors send a signal to the brain. One particularly important nerve, the vagus nerve, is activated. The activation of this nerve has a number of interesting effects. It results in a decrease in blood pressure and heart rate. In addition, touch reduces levels of cortisol (a hormone involved in the stress response) and increases the release of oxytocin which, as we have seen, promotes feelings of trust, bonding and devotion. Touch effectively puts us in a state of reduced stress and immerses us in the emotion of love.

In western culture it is not uncommon for an infant to be separated post birth, particularly with a medicalised birth. Skin-to-skin contact between the mother and baby should occur at the moment of birth, and the naked baby should be placed on the mother's bare chest, covered with a warm blanket. It has been observed in mammalian neuroscientific studies that 'the intimate contact inherent in this place (habitat) evokes neurobehaviors ensuring fulfillment of basic biological needs'[47] and that 'this time may represent a psychophysiologically 'sensitive period' for programming future physiology and behavior.' This sensitive period is a window of opportunity for the mother and baby to experience the most magical period of love and bonding.

The effect of the skin-to-skin contact is not limited to the baby. Research has shown that skin-to-skin contact can reduce the risk of postpartum depression. In one particular study, mothers gave about 5 hours per day of skin-to-skin contact with their babies in the first week following birth and then more than 2 hours per day until the infants were age one month. The mothers in the skin-to-skin contact group, compared to mothers in the control group, who provided little or no skin-to-skin contact, had lower scores on the depression scales when the infants were one week old. In addition, the mothers in the skin-to-skin group had a reduction in salivary cortisol in their infants' first month. This study demonstrates the positive effect of skin-to-skin contact between the mother and baby in the postpartum period.[48]

Touch not only has these direct physiological benefits to the mother and baby, but it also provides the perfect situation to begin eye-to-eye contact and encourages emotionally positive actions such as cuddling, hugging and kissing. It also has been shown to promote breastfeeding.[49] There are many other benefits of skin-to-skin contact regarding the maintenance of optimal physiological balance for the baby, including regulation of heart rate, respiration and temperature, to name a few.[50] Babies who experience skin-to-skin contact have reduced crying and fall asleep more easily.[51] The countless physiological benefits aside, it just feels wondrous, natural, and instinctual. It is how post birth was meant to feel – prolonged periods of immersing in the delight of bonding.

Continuation of Bonding and Attachment

Establishing effective bonding with the baby requires extended periods of contact.[52] I outline the main ways in which we can continue this bonding below. It includes breastfeeding/attentive bottle-feeding, cosleeping and touch (in the form of infant massage).

Breastfeeding

The benefits of breastfeeding are extensive[53], and the importance of promoting the initiation and continuation of breastfeeding has come to the forefront of postpartum care. Breastfeeding promotes bonding between the mother and baby, through the undivided attention given to the baby whilst being awash in oxytocin. It also keeps the baby in close proximity to the mother's heartbeat, which reduces the amount of stress hormones in the baby. This experience will promote a healthy bond of trust and love. The most important aspect of feeding a baby, whether by breast or bottle, is ensuring undivided attention and love, since the pattern of predictable care and attention will effectively program the baby into a relationship of trust and love with the mother, and in the case of bottle-feeding, the other parent as well.

The World Health Organization recommends exclusive breastfeeding for babies to 6 months of age, and thereafter for breastfeeding to continue alongside suitable complementary foods for up to 2 years and beyond.[54] Despite these recommendations the rates of breastfeeding in Australia are substandard. In fact, although 96% of mothers are able to initiate breastfeeding, only 15% are still being exclusively breastfed at 5 months of age.[55]

Breastfeeding benefits both the mother and the baby.[56] The baby receives the ideal food that is rich in antibodies. These antibodies act to protect the baby from many childhood illnesses. In addition, breastfeeding promotes good health later in life, with research showing that babies who were breastfed are less likely to be overweight or obese later in life, and have lower rates of type II diabetes. They have also been shown to perform higher on intelligence tests. Mothers benefit by having reduced rates of breast and ovarian cancer, type II diabetes, and postpartum depression.

It is evident that breastfeeding is highly beneficial to the mother and baby, but we must ask ourselves why there are such low rates of breastfeeding? It is imperative that women receive the support necessary to implement and sustain breastfeeding. This should not only take place at home, but also at a community level, and most certainly workplaces should provide women who return to work with the ability to express milk.

The long-term positive effects of breastfeeding for mother and baby mean it is something that should not be treated as an inconvenience by society. This is a fundamental part of early attachment which sows the seeds of later good health, and is highly beneficial to the baby's and mother's immediate mental and physical health.

It is beyond time that this important element of human attachment and bonding is prioritised and supported as a vital element of postnatal care, within the home, by society, and by governments at large. Even medical professionals have been found to be woefully inept at providing advice and support for breastfeeding mothers. This demonstrates a lack of training opportunities for medical professionals, particularly GPs, who often find themselves as the first port of call for a mother who needs advice on breastfeeding.[57]

When breastfeeding is unable to be initiated, the mother and father can experience bonding through bottle-feeding. The baby is still held close to the heart, experiences the love, eye contact, smells, warmth and undivided attention; all of which are pivotal to bonding.[58]

Mother-infant cosleeping

> *'…we must accept that the modern Western custom of an independent childhood sleeping pattern is unique and exceedingly rare among contemporary and past world cultures.'*[59]

Cosleeping is any situation where the caregiver and infant or child are within sensory range of each other. This gives the caregiver and the infant the ability to respond to the sensory cues of each other. Therefore, this definition includes room sharing and also the more intimate bed sharing. Solitary sleeping, on the other hand, is the practice whereby the baby sleeps in a separate room to the parent or caregiver.

There are two equally important perspectives that must be addressed to determine the safety and advantages of cosleeping. Firstly, we must explore the most recent research conducted into these practices, and secondly, we must view these practices through the lens of the anthropologist and the biological heritage of the baby.

Mother-infant cosleeping has been practiced since time immemorial, and is the most successful way of infant sleeping – it has ensured the survival of the human race. It has only been a recent phenomenon in a select group of people (Western and industrialised nations) to separate the infant from the mother in a solitary sleeping arrangement. It is also important to recognise that SIDS (Sudden Infant Death Syndrome) is also a phenomenon unique to Western civilisation – to which around 600,000 babies have been lost.[60]

We exist within a rapidly changing society and culture; we can't deny the pressures and expectations that modern living imposes on us. There is mounting pressure on mothers to become increasingly self-sufficient and independent, and these are qualities that we are therefore expecting of our infants, even though this is at odds with what infants actually are; that is, highly dependent.[61] Our rapidly changing culture is finding itself in conflict with our innate physiology, which evolved under very different conditions.

The effects of our ever-changing world on our physiology are evident on many levels, but are most obvious when we observe the multitude of lifestyle diseases in our adult population. It also raises the highly important question of whether we should alter the traditional methods of child rearing for the sake of convenience and the expedience of modern living. We need to ask whether recent western social values have been prioritised over the biological heritage of our infants and children, and if so, what are the long-term consequences, and is this sacrifice worth it? [62]

In the world of the infant, the 'mother is the environment.'[63] Dr James McKenna, biological anthropologist and leading authority on mother-infant cosleeping, eloquently discusses the how the sensory interaction of the infant and mother is absolutely important in that it regulates the behavioural and physiological microenvironment of the child. The exchange of touch, smell, sound, taste and movement is imperative to the baby's ability to regulate its own environment.[64] Babies who cosleep maintain lighter sleep and rouse more frequently, which protects the babies from apnoeas (the temporary cessation of breathing). They therefore maintain higher levels of oxygenation. The baby is also able to maintain the right body temperature. Cosleeping or bed sharing also encourages more regular breastfeeding. Babies are not physiologically designed to exist as independent from the mother.

Cosleeping or bed sharing safely

> *'A baby's cry is precisely as serious as it sounds.'*
>
> Jean Leidloff
> **Author of *The Continuum Concept, In Search of Happiness Lost***

There are of course safe and unsafe practices with either cosleeping or bed sharing. If practiced safely, it is undoubtedly a secure and most physiologically sound form of infant sleep. There are a number of things to keep in mind when deciding to cosleep or bed share with your baby.

- Parents should not smoke.

- Parents should not be under the influence of any drugs including alcohol.
- The baby should be laying prone (on their back).
- Heavy duvets should be avoided and never over the head of the baby.
- There should be no gaps into which the baby can fall.
- Ideally there should not be other children in the bed.
- It is not recommended to bed share with bottle-fed infants. As an alternative, it is recommended they sleep on a different surface, but in close proximity to the mother. This is because mothers who bottle feed their babies do not have the same responsive parenting at night as breastfeeding mothers do.
- Couch sleeping is never safe.

It becomes clear from assessing the research, our biological imperatives and our gut instincts regarding what feels right, that cosleeping or bed sharing with your baby, if done sensibly and safely, has the best outcomes for mother and child. Not only is the baby more likely to be breastfed (and more regularly), the stimulation of the senses increases brain growth, they are within an environment which feels safe and secure and their physiology is kept within a range that promotes well-being.

It is fundamental that parents are aware of their rights to cosleep and bedshare with their babies and children, and that they have access to the information and support to undertake this tremendously satisfying experience. After all, it is how we are biologically designed to care for our infants and children.[ii]

Infant massage

'Being touched and caressed, being massaged, is food for the infant; food as necessary as minerals, vitamins and proteins.'

Frederick Leboyer M.D.
French Obstetrician and Author

Baby massage is a practice that has been undertaken for thousands of years in some cultures. People from the Western world are becoming more aware of this practice as an enjoyable way to bond with their infant or child. Touch is the first sense to develop in the foetus. It is the most primitive sense and involves the largest organ in our body – the skin.[65] Infants in the first few months of life predominantly rely on this sense to learn about the environment and the emotions of the people around them.[66]

It is well known that babies who do not receive loving touch can develop many physical and psychological issues – such as 'small body stature, altered brain function, and the reproduction of stereotypic movements such as rocking or arm flapping.'[67] It is not only beneficial, but also imperative that an infant or child receives caring touch from their mother, father or primary carer, and massage is a beautiful expression of this loving touch.

The benefits of massage to the baby are well documented. Physically, the baby will benefit from improved sleep, improved cognitive development

---

[ii] I highly recommend visiting Dr James McKenna's website which has comprehensive information regarding cosleeping and bed sharing. http://cosleeping.nd.edu/

and reduced symptoms of colic. Psychologically the baby will benefit from the bonding that takes place within this loving, relaxed environment with a responsive and attentive parent or carer. A number of studies have shown the benefits of infant massage for preterm infants as well, one being weight gain. Stimulation of the vagus nerve regulates gastric motility and helps with digestion of food, increasing the availability of nutrients. Additionally, the stimulation of the vagus nerve increases the release of insulin, which leads to release of insulin-like-growth-factor-1 (IGF-1), which regulates growth.[68]

As well as encouraging attachment between the mother (or primary carer) and child, studies have shown that infant massage results in more positive attitudes of mothers towards their experience of motherhood.[69] Infant massage also has a positive effect on mothers with postnatal depression. In one study, after undertaking the practice of infant massage for one year, mothers with postnatal depression had non-depressed levels of sensitivity of interaction with their babies.[70] The beautiful, relaxing experience of infant massage is an enjoyable way of promoting the precious experience of bonding between the parent and infant.

Important information for infant massage

- Massage should only be started after the navel has healed and the baby has gained some strength. This is at around 4 weeks.
- A good time of day to do infant massage is just before bath time in the evening, as it will encourage a relaxing sleep.
- Choose a time when the baby is content and happy and only do the massage if the baby is untroubled while you are doing it.

- Make sure the environment is warm, and the oil is warm (body temperature). Make sure you test the warmth of the oil before putting it on the baby.
- This is a special time of communication and attention to your baby. Make sure there are no other distractions. It is lovely to sing or talk with your baby during this time.
- The best oils to use are organic. Traditionally coconut or sesame oil have been used. Examples of other oils that can be used are almond or jojoba. You may want to patch test the oil on the baby before using it (apply the oil to the inside of the babies arm and wait 24 hours to see if there is any reaction). Make sure you do not use mineral-based oils or oils which contain essential oils or oils that contain perfumes.

Striving to Meet Human Potential

At every stage of a child's development, it is profoundly important that we *maintain the progression of meaningful and loving bonding between parent and child*. This, I maintain, is the common thread that binds each of the significant stages (conception, pregnancy, childbirth and early childhood). The process of bonding in the early stages of child creation has an effect on the future capacity of the child to love oneself, love others, and accept love. This can be recognised as being the single most important capability of any human being. Without the capacity to experience or express love, life is meaningless.

Truth 1 Summary

- *Biological expectations* are certain nutritional, physical and psychological needs that all babies are born with to ensure their safe and healthy development into adulthood.
- Human babies are born the most immature and helpless of any living creature on this planet.
- The most fundamental biological expectations of a baby include:
  - Skin-to-skin contact after birth
  - Physical contact
  - Being responded to when in need
  - Child sleeping in close proximity with the mother/father or carer
  - Breastfeeding or bottle-feeding as per the baby's demand
- Meeting biological expectations ensures healthy attachment (bonding).
- We must maintain the progression of meaningful and loving bonding between the parent/carer and child.
- You cannot over-attach with the child.
- Healthy attachment is vital for healthy psychological development.
- Children are biologically hardwired to attach, and will attach to those spending the most time with them.
- If you spend lengthy periods of the day apart from your child, it is wise to commit time and effort to re-attach with the child after each period of separation.
- The quantity of time you spend with your child matters.

- Attachment occurs at the stages of conception, pregnancy, birth and beyond and there are various ways in which we can promote attachment at each of these stages.

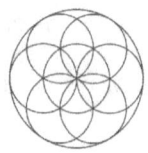

TRUTH TWO

*What We Inscribe In The Child's Mind
Will Echo Throughout Their Lifetime*

Sowing the Seeds of Change

> *'Enlightened collectives will fulfill an important function in the arising of the new consciousness. Just as egoic collectives pull you into unconsciousness and suffering, the enlightened collective can be a vortex for consciousness that will accelerate the planetary shift.'*[71]
>
> Eckhart Tolle
> **Spiritual Teacher, Author**

Our children give us the opportunity to influence the trajectory of humanity in a positive way. By nurturing and encouraging the development of expansive minds, love and compassion, we are creating a potential for the blossoming of greatness in the future. As parents, one of our most powerful impacts on humanity could be the children that we are raising, and the way in which they will steer our world.

Through the creation of these 'enlightened collectives' we may witness change rapidly and effectively. We must give our young children the opportunity to develop the wisdom and spiritual awareness they will need to confront the challenges of the future. Are we creating the space, attention, foundations for good health and love that our children require to meet the potential they were gifted at conception? And what can we do to foster these qualities in our upcoming generations?

Shifting Focus

Our culture is primarily based on the Newtonian concept of reality – that matter is foremost. As a result, many of us do not look beyond that which exists in the physical plane. Our children, as a product of this culture, are being raised with a strong identification with the world of form. Developing a balance between the world of form, and that which exists on a deeper level is a powerful way to cultivate psychologically balanced individuals.

Awareness

Awareness, in a spiritual sense, is the ability to be conscious of one's thoughts and feelings. A human being is basically the combination of their perceptions, thoughts and emotions. The subtle differences in these elements make us so very different from one another. Self-awareness or self-knowing is examining yourself from the background of your past, but in the present moment. It is an awareness of what is actually taking place, rather than what you *think* you are or what you *should* be.

Self-awareness could also be described as being consciously aware of how your ego is controlling your thoughts, feelings or actions at that time.

L. Krishnamurti eloquently described this process in an extract from a talk in 1976, where he stated that observation can only take place in the now and should take place without condemnation or judgment – we are to let the perception, thought or emotion flower, then disappear. And in doing that, one becomes a light to oneself.

The development of awareness in the minds of children will pave the path for the creation of these 'enlightened collectives'. Awareness can enable children to identify with their *essence* rather than with a limited *form* identity. This will result in true success. If we as parents, carers and teachers can precipitate the acknowledgement of this transcendent dimension of consciousness in children, it would undoubtedly result in a quickening of evolution of consciousness on the planet, and an alignment with universal consciousness.

What can we practice with our children to develop their awareness?

Developing awareness in children essentially involves helping them recognise and acknowledge their emotions as they arise. A simple practice would be to observe these emotions like a blossoming flower, and watch it pass. One can only imagine the positive implications in a child's life by learning this process.

One of the most important processes is to allow the child to feel emotion, and to be present with the child in the moment of this emotional expression. Our instinctive reaction to a child conveying emotion is to reason with them as to why they shouldn't feel that way, or in more extreme situations make ourselves physically and emotionally unavailable to them. This is practiced in certain techniques such as 'time out'. What the child needs is to feel the presence of a caring adult and the time to allow them to express their emotion.

Repressing emotions is a very common practice among the adult population, and this is likely to be a result of a culture that is uncomfortable with emotional expression and a childhood that was littered with the message that 'emotional vulnerability is not welcome here.' The process of being present for a child during their most vulnerable moments creates a great depth of attachment. A child should *always* feel that they are worthy of love, and should not have the fear of love being withdrawn, especially as a result of the emotions they are experiencing.

What a gift to a child if awareness were to be integrated into every aspect of their education. What a gift to assist a child with identifying and dealing with emotions at the time they arise. As the child grows, they will be able to cope with the various experiences of life with a calmness and serenity that accompanies awareness, rather than riding the tumultuous roller coaster of knee-jerk emotional reactions to countless challenging situations.

It is impossible to avoid suffering in this world; it is inevitable. But as the child grows, with an understanding of how to practice awareness, they will be better equipped to deal with whatever challenges arise. This process of developing self-awareness in children is not only a gift to the child but to the whole of humanity.

As parents we must provide many moments of presence for our children. Bringing these moments of consciousness is imperative to creating a harmonious relationship with them. We need to move away from being trapped in the process of continuously doing and thinking, and instead step into a space of attention towards our children.

Introducing small moments of focused attention to the needs of the child can make a difference. Our spiritual challenge as parents is to be able to create these moments of stillness and presence. It can be a challenge to do this, as it is sometimes very difficult to avoid reacting with anger and resistance towards a child who is not working with your plan of how the day should unfold. Children provide us with the ultimate opportunity to exercise this fundamental spiritual practice of presence. And for this we should be grateful.

Consistently responding to the child

The main way to develop healthy attachment is by responding to the needs of the child in a loving and compassionate way. With consistent and predictable responses to their expression of need, over time, the child is able to regulate their own emotions. We must remind ourselves that the young child's primary form of communication is crying, and that responding to their needs will reinforce their emotional development and strengthen the attachment process.

By doing this we will hardwire into the brain of the child the knowledge that 'If I cry out, someone is there to respond to my needs, and I am loved'. Responding to the needs of the child enhances their resilience and independence later in life.[72] You can never show a child too much love. There is no better foundation on which to build our future society than a collective belief that they are loved, and that people will listen and are there to help when they are in need.

Mindfulness practices for children

Introducing meditation or mindfulness practices is a lovely way to develop the skill of practicing presence in children. It does not need to be a complex or elaborate process, rather a time of quiet reflection within. Building the skill of turning the attention from without to within is a practice that can be used throughout life. This process also aids emotional regulation and cognitive focus. Mindfulness practices are particularly useful for children who are experiencing stress and may aid children who are experiencing behavioural difficulties. Clarity is a source of power and mindfulness creates clarity of thought.

Nourishing the Brain With Love

> *'The true character of a society is revealed in how it treats its children.'*
>
> Nelson Mandela
> **South African Anti-Apartheid Revolutionary**

The brain of a baby undergoes rapid development over the first several years of life. The extended infancy period is a reflection of the vast amount of information that is incorporated into the brain post birth.[73] The human brain takes close to 25 years to reach full maturity; the longest of any mammal.[74] By eighteen months of age the child's brain will weigh close to two thirds of its adult weight.[75] This rapid brain development is a result of the experiences – emotional, sensory, motor and cognitive – of the child.[76]

This period in a child's development is one of enormous potential, but also requires great care as it represents a time of supercharged hardwiring of the brain. We must treat this timeframe with utmost respect and attempt to provide an environment that maximises the healthy development of the brain. Those people who have primary contact with the child in these early years are effectively engineering their mind.

The conscious and subconscious mind

Human consciousness exists essentially as a duality – the two primary aspects being the subconscious and the conscious minds. Understanding the dual nature of the human mind is essential to appreciating behaviour, and particularly, the way in which it shapes our external, objective experiences. In its infancy, the human brain undergoes a phenomenally rapid download for the purposes of survival. This will be a program of not only a skill set, but also a belief set, about how and where they fit in the scheme of things.

It is imperative that we understand this aspect of child psychology. Although the content may seem heavy, it is worth every iota of effort to grasp it, for this really is the foundation of your child's belief system later in life. It heavily influences your child's 'self-talk' as an adult – and as we know, that is what can make all the difference.

Gaining an understanding of how our mind works enables us to begin appreciating how and why we behave and react to external stimulus in the way that we do. It makes us ponder the extent to which we, as parents, are responsible for the 'programming' of our children's minds, and the resulting lifelong mindsets.

Our responsibility to understand this process is pivotal, if we are to raise human beings that are of a healthy mentality. This will directly translate into a tangible improvement in the world around us. Parents and carers have the ability to contribute to significant and much-needed change in the world through the children we raise, as they 'are the living messages we send to a time we will not see.'[77]

To understand the human mind, it is most useful to think of it in terms of the conscious, subconscious and unconscious – all of which are interrelated. Sigmund Freud made this concept popular and from his theories, an illustrative metaphor of the 'Freudian iceberg' was born.[78]

Conscious mind (or the ego)

This is depicted as the tip of the iceberg, visible above the surface of the water. This is our rational mind. These are the mental processes over which we exercise free will. It only occupies about 10% of the brain's capacity. It is our concept of 'self' and the voice of our thoughts.

Subconscious mind (or the preconscious)

The subconscious mind dwells just below the level of consciousness. In contrast to the unconscious mind, the subconscious thoughts and feelings can be easily brought to consciousness. This, together with our unconscious mind, drives our behaviour.

Unconscious mind

The unconscious mind determines our beliefs, habits and behaviours. This aspect of the mind is, according to Freud, the most important determining factor of human behaviour. It stores our memories and past experiences that are inaccessible to our conscious mind. The subconscious and unconscious minds make up 90% of our brain's capacity and together, form the predominant, submerged part of the iceberg.

How are these three aspects of the mind related?

The unconscious mind communicates to your conscious mind through your subconscious. Together, these three facets of the mind create our perception of reality. As we now understand how these three aspects of the mind are intrinsically linked and the predominance of our subconscious and unconscious minds, it begs the question, how are our subconscious and unconscious minds *programmed*? They are, after all, effectively determining our perceptions of our world and therefore creating our reality. In fact, Dr Bruce Lipton in his book *The Biology of Belief*, explains that the subconscious mind processes some 20,000,000 environmental stimuli per second compared to the 40 environmental stimuli processed by the conscious mind in the same second.[79]

Programming the subconscious mind

The effect of the programming in our subconscious mind cannot be overstated. This program affects all aspects of our life - our beliefs, our limitations, and even our physiology and health. Once the subconscious is hardwired it remains fixed, unless we go through the arduous effort of rewiring. In order to understand when and how the subconscious and unconscious minds are programmed, we need to look at the brain state of children up to the formation of the conscious mind.

The human brain is designed to retain a huge quantity of information in the early years of life to ensure rapid learning for survival. This information is integrated into the subconscious and unconscious minds. At various stages of a child's development it has been observed that different brain wave activity predominates.

Brain waves are electrical voltages in the brain and measure a few millionths of a volt. In any given moment there will be a combination of various types of brain waves detectable, but we can observe what the predominant brain waves are through measurements made with an EEG (electroencephalogram). There are five main types of brain waves which can represent different mind states:

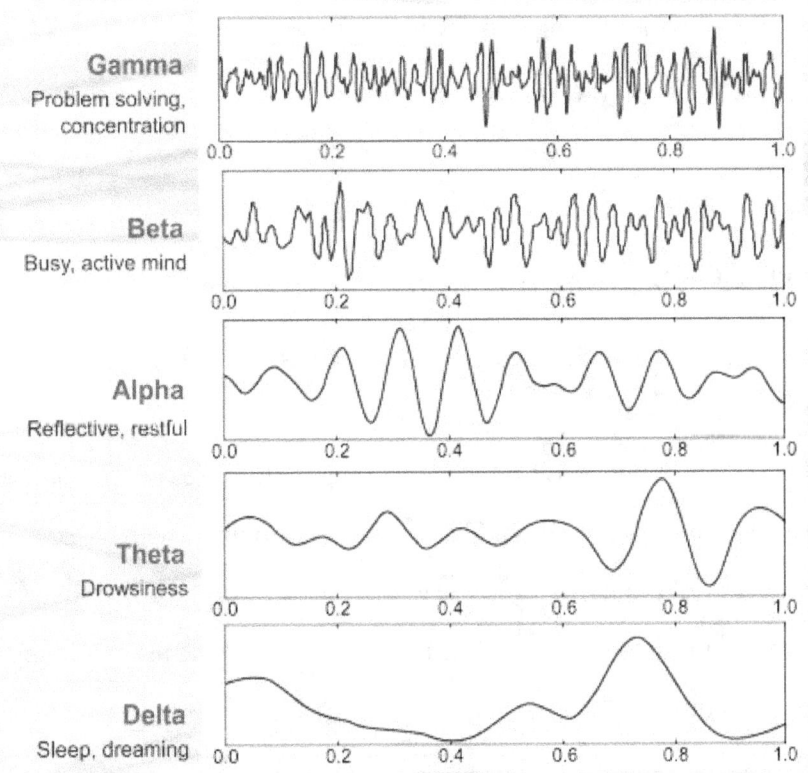

Diagram 4: Examples of alpha, beta, theta, delta and gamma brain wave forms.[80]

The brain wave states of children develop and evolve over time into adulthood. Let us look at each stage: (See Table 2)

Birth – 2 years

Delta waves predominate in children up to the age of around 2 years. They have the slowest EEG activity (0.5 – 4 Hz). Delta waves in adults are involved in deep sleep, and very deep relaxation.

Around 2 – 6 years

The child begins to spend more time in the *Theta* state (4 - 8Hz). The theta state is experienced in adults when drifting off to sleep or just waking up. It is also predominant during hypnosis, and meditation. During experiences of being 'in the zone' theta waves predominate. From the age of around 2 – 6 years children are living in a world of imagination. Creativity is rich during this period.

Around 6 – 12 years

There is an increased presence of *Alpha* waves (8 - 12 Hz). The alpha state is one of being relaxed and alert, and in adults occurs during meditation, lighter states of relaxation and daydreaming. At this age the conscious mind is not dominant, so there is still a window of opportunity to influence your child's view of themselves and the world through your positive suggestions. However, during this time period, the impact of outside programming does begin to reduce.

12 years and beyond

During this time there is an increase in the periods of *Beta* waves (12-35 Hz). By the time the child reaches adolescence, the subconscious mind is filled with the information necessary for survival and most of the self-perceptions and beliefs they will carry with them into adulthood.

AGE	PREDOMINANT BRAINWAVE	FREQUENCY	WHAT IS TAKING PLACE	WHAT YOU CAN DO
BIRTH – 2 YEARS	DELTA	0.5 – 4 Hz	Very deep relaxation	Engage the infant/child in conversation
AROUND 2 – 6 YEARS	THETA	4-8 Hz	There is an increase in creative thinking and imagination	Encourage and stimulate your child's creativity
AROUND 6 – 12 YEARS	ALPHA	8-12 Hz	Mind is in a relaxed and alert state	Be mindful of what you suggest to the child as it will become part of their beliefs about themselves and the world around them
12 YEARS AND BEYOND	ALPHA with increased periods of BETA	12-35 Hz	The conscious mind is now dominant	Be a support in assisting the child to become consciously aware of their emotions and behaviour

Table 2: Summary of the brainwaves present at various ages.[81] Looking at the predominant or evolving brain waves helps us understand what is taking place in the child's mind and what we can do to assist them at that time.

Rapid Download

During the period of birth to around 6 years, children are able to download a phenomenal quantity of information about the environment around them. Hypnotherapists aim to get people into the delta or theta brain wave state because of their increased suggestibility. Children absorb, in an unfiltered manner, the beliefs and behaviour of those in their environment; most frequently their parents. Children at this age do not have a developed analytical (conscious) mind through which to filter input during these early years. It is as though they are in a hypnotic state, hardwiring the suggestions and behaviours of those around them into their brains, as *truths*.

As a parent myself, on initially reading this as explained by Dr Bruce Lipton in his book *The Biology of Belief*, I felt that I had come across one of the most pivotal and fundamentally important pieces of information on parenting – we are effectively programming the minds of our children. We are therefore largely responsible for the beliefs, habits, and self-perceptions of our children. What an incredibly powerful, yet daunting acknowledgment.

This information raises a number of issues that cannot be ignored. It requires us to make a very close and careful assessment of who is programming the minds of our children. It becomes the parents' responsibility to acknowledge who the child is spending the predominant time of their waking life with. We need to ask ourselves whether or not we feel confident that the subtle, powerful and continuous messages they are getting are ones we are comfortable with them carrying potentially for a lifetime. If you are not programming the minds of your children, who is? It really is as simple as that.

In addition, one has to realise that reprogramming your subconscious mind as an adult (if required) is not an easy task, and requires a lot of effort (although it is possible)[iii]. Many adults carry with them the burden of a childhood that has perhaps not resulted in an ideal programming of the subconscious. As the subconscious is responsible for much of our automatic behaviour, we begin to understand the far-reaching ramifications.

[iii] Works by Dr Joseph Dispenza and Dr Bruce Lipton are useful for information on this subject.

We have the potential to create a whole new wave of empowered children who will be the ones to tackle the issues of the future - an 'enlightened collective' who will push the boundaries of possibility and healing of humanity. This will be a healing from the foundations. Frederick Douglass expressed this eloquently when he said, 'It is easier to build strong children than to repair broken men.'

Who's the boss? Conscious decision-making and the unconscious mind

A hard concept to fathom is that contrary to what we believe, our unconscious mind has already made a decision seconds before it enters our conscious awareness. Many processes occur in our brain at an unconscious level for mundane and routine tasks - this is to prevent overload. Contrary to our prior belief that decision-making is a conscious process, researchers have found that the decision-making process is largely undertaken by the unconscious mind. This means that you have actually already made a decision prior to the point of reaching the 'decision' in your conscious mind.

The findings of research in this area challenge our strongly held belief of free will and conscious control of our decision-making. As quoted by the researchers: 'The impression that we are able to freely choose between different possible causes of action is fundamental to our mental life. However, it has been suggested that this subjective experience of freedom is no more than an illusion and that our actions are initiated by unconscious mental processes long before we become aware of our intention to act.'[82]

In this study, participants were asked to choose whether to press a button in their right or left hand. They could take as much time as they wanted to make the decision, but had to remember at what point they made the decision. The findings were astounding: '...two specific regions in the frontal and parietal cortex of the human brain had considerable information that predicted the outcome of a motor decision the subject had not yet consciously made. This suggests that when the subject's decision reached awareness it had been influenced by unconscious brain activity for up to 10 seconds...'[83] Further research is yet to be conducted to uncover where the final decision is made and whether or not these decisions can be reversed.

This research illustrates that our unconscious mind prepares our decisions. The way in which our subconscious and unconscious minds are wired directly affects the decisions that we make, and this research suggests that the conscious mind has less input in this process than we previous believed.

The expeditious encoding of information into the subconscious mind of the child matters for this reason. It can ultimately affect the decision making process and therefore many of the choices that the child makes later in their adult life. It is with this consideration in mind that we should approach parenting young children with care and mindfulness of the belief set we are strongly influencing and moulding.

Door to the Subconscious Mind

'In a dream, in a vision of the night, when deep sleep falleth upon men, in slumbering upon the bed; then he openeth the ears of men and sealeth their instruction.'

Book of Job 33

A beautiful time of day with your child is the time before they drift off to sleep. I think of this time as a period of heightened suggestibility. It is the perfect opportunity to tell the child that they are loved, confident, intelligent, healthy and strong. I love to tell my daughters that I am always there to listen for them, and that they can tell me anything without judgment. You can use this time to express to them those qualities you would like integrated into their minds. It is such a calming and precious way to spend time with your children. This is a very powerful time as the child is in a heightened state of suggestibility. Use this time to create a positive mindset in the child, and to appease any concerns.

We must remind ourselves that when we are influencing the programming of our child's subconscious mind, we are not only programming that one mind, but we are also influencing the collective consciousness of humanity. What an incredible gift this is for mankind.

Statements of love for your child

You are so loved
You are beautiful, strong and healthy
I am so grateful that you are my child
What you have to say matters and I am here to listen to you
I am always here to listen to how you are feeling
You have so many incredible qualities to give to this world
You can achieve so much in this world
I look forward to the many wonderful things we will experience together
You have excitement and adventure to look forward to in this life
I am proud of who you are
Your family and friends love and cherish you

Truth 2 Summary

- Awareness in a spiritual sense is the ability to be conscious of one's thoughts and feelings.
- Developing awareness in children is a way of helping them identify with their essence rather than purely with their form identity.
- To develop awareness in children, we must assist them in recognising their emotions as they arise.
- Responding to the needs of the child in a loving and compassionate way helps them develop the ability to regulate their own emotions.
- Understanding the predominant brain waves at various stages in a child's development enables us, as parents and carers, to determine what we can do to assist them as they grow.
- We have an enormous impact on the programming of the subconscious mind of children as they are experiencing rapid learning during childhood.

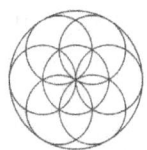

TRUTH THREE

*Parents are Genetic
Engineers – Epigenetics and
Engineering the Future*

Epigenetics

Epigenetics is a relatively new area of science that is providing us with concrete evidence as to the long-term effects of various approaches to conception and pregnancy, childbirth and parenting. Continued scientific research has helped us understand the delicate interplay between our genetic expression and our environmental influences. The knowledge we have gained in this area of science brings to our attention the importance of honouring and nurturing the period of childhood.

Dr Bruce Lipton's book *The Biology of Belief* [84], explains the concept of Epigenetics, and how it can be a tool to develop greatness. We are essentially free to exhibit and live to the full potential of our DNA, which is less restrictive than we may have previously believed.

For those of us who need a strong scientific reason to adopt a particular approach to conception, pregnancy, birth and child raising, epigenetics provides us with growing evidence. Our lifestyle choices and our mental frame directly influence the humans that we create and epigenetics explains why.

Epigenetics as a Reason to Honour Child Creation

What is epigenetics?

Genetic determinism is the belief that one's heredity or genetic makeup is fixed from the time of birth, unperturbed by the influence of the external environment. This belief has been challenged by the study of epigenetics. This field of study emerged in the 1940s and is 'one of the most rapidly developing fields of biological research.'[85] There is now evidence that both our environment and our experience can alter our genetic expression.[86] We are all familiar with the concept of nature versus nurture. Epigenetics is now seen as a third area of contemplation in regards to our genetic expression.

I recently read an eloquent analogy that helps us understand epigenetics. If the DNA is the unique 'song of you', the epigenome can be viewed as the 'audio engineers' that can change the way that song is played (the volume, the quality, adding or removal of certain instruments). In the same way, the reading of our DNA can be changed by the epigenome.[87] Throughout life, orchestrated chemical reactions can affect our genome by either activating or deactivating various parts at various times and in various locations on our DNA. Epigenetics describes the process of these chemical reactions and what influences them.

In every cell we have DNA that encodes for genetic instruction and stores all of our biological information. The DNA is wrapped tightly so it can fit inside the cell; keep in mind that if we were to unravel the DNA, it would be 6 foot long. The ability of the cell to 'read' the DNA is essential for healthy expression of the genes. This is where epigenetics plays a pivotal role.

Epigenetic markers are a set of instructions that sit on top of your DNA and histones (histones are proteins that are responsible for DNA packaging and are involved in the controlling the expression of genes). As the word itself suggests – 'epi' meaning on top of and 'genetics' meaning your genes. Epigenetic markers are chemical tags that influence whether the gene should compress or unravel to allow the cell to read the instructions on the DNA. This epigenetic instruction essentially dictates which genes are 'switched on' and which genes are 'switched off'. This determines our biological expression, and therefore governs what level of our personal human potential we reach.

Epigenetics is the link between our heredity and our environmental influences, and it shapes not only our health, but also our personality and behaviour.[88] In addition, the epigenetic inheritance system enables the parents to 'transfer' information to their offspring regarding the environment in which they exist. In this way, parents can be described as 'genetic engineers' of their children, as suggested by Dr Bruce Lipton in his book *The Biology of Belief*.[89]

The laying down of epigenetic markers

It is important to know that this epigenetic information is established at a greater level during embryonic development. Epigenetic markers are not only influenced by the surrounding cells, but also by the environment surrounding the developing embryo. These not only include what the mother is putting into her body such as food, beverages, chemicals, medications, supplements; but also the levels of stress and the mental state that the mother is in, all of which is translated into a myriad of chemical signals in the shared blood stream.

The signals that the foetus receives during this sensitive time will affect their epigenetic markings and therefore their genetic expression. The actions of the mother during pregnancy can have far reaching consequences for the health and well-being of the offspring. And as I will discuss below, even the actions of the mother and father prior to conception, and the actions of previous generations can influence the outcomes of later generations through epigenetic imprinting, like ghosts from the past.

The epigenetic markers that are laid down in great amounts during embryonic development are effectively a way of preparing the foetus for the type of environment that the parents are experiencing in the external world. The environment the parents are in, and the emotional reactions to those experiences, are affecting the genetic expression of the child. The experiences of the parents can become impressions on the genetics of the foetus.

From a survival point of view, this makes perfect sense. It is paramount to the survival of the child that they are prepared for the environment in which they will be born. Nature has allowed certain flexibility for the development of the child depending on the external environment. In certain instances this information can be adaptive, but in other cases it can pose significant disharmony for the child. One such example is the effect of stress on the unborn infant.

Stress, the unborn infant and epigenetics

The particular case of stress in the mother and the effect on the unborn infant's epigenome is interesting to consider, as stress is a pervasive emotion in today's society. It has been believed, since time immemorial, that the emotional state of the mother influences the health of the unborn child. There is now mounting evidence that this is no longer an old wives' tale.

We must make the distinction between chronic stress and acute stress (which our bodies are well-equipped to handle). Chronic stress is continual, unrelenting and over time can disrupt physical and mental well-being. There are a number of chemicals produced in the body in response to stress, cortisol and adrenaline being two of the more familiar ones. In reality, the process is much more complex and involves many other substances which interact with each other.

As we have previously discussed, these stress chemicals not only affect the mother, but literally traverse through the placenta and bathe the growing foetus. These chemicals signal the foetus to grow and develop in a way that will maximise its chances of survival in a world that the mother perceives as adverse.

It is now known that women who experience stress during pregnancy are at a greater risk of preterm birth, smaller birth weight and length of babies, and those same babies are at a greater risk of asthma, allergies, and infectious diseases. Not only is the physical health of the child at risk, but the mental health and cognition of the child is also compromised, with increased fussiness and temperamental problems, and lower scores on measures of mental development. It has even been proposed that 'prenatal stress, through the generation of epigenetic alterations, becomes one of the most powerful influences on mental health in later life.'[90]

The effects of maternal stress through changes in the epigenome of the foetus can impact the health of the endocrine and brain development not only of the foetus but across several generations.[91] It is now clear that being cognisant of the effects of stress on the growing foetus and on future generations is vital in supporting healthy development in the present and in the future. Studies in epigenetics demonstrate that not only is the foetus affected by the mother's molecules of emotions, but also by ancestral epigenetic signatures.

This is an example of the mind's power to affect the body, and also future outcomes. This occurs purely because stress (our interpretation of the environment) creates a cascade of chemical changes in the body that flow though the blood stream, which is shared with the foetus. Not only are we moulding the development of the foetus through the chemical mixture in which the growing baby is awash, but also potentially our future lineage.

External environmental influences on the unborn infant

Through the study of epigenetics, we are also beginning to unearth not only how an individual's environment can affect their metabolism, but also how the metabolism is affected by the environment experienced by the parents. We are now learning that women who eat poor diets are more likely to produce offspring who will develop obesity or type II diabetes.[92] The adverse intrauterine environment increases the risk of the development of disease later in life. Although a majority of studies focus on the effect of maternal health on the unborn child, there is mounting evidence that paternal exposure to poor diet can also have an effect on the subsequent development of metabolic disorders in their offspring.[93]

Trans-generational Inheritance of Epigenetic Markers

An interesting area of study is the multigenerational transmission of epigenetic markers. That is, the experiences of your grandparents can be transmitted to you through epigenetic markings. It has been shown in a Swedish population that over nutrition of the grandparents during their early childhood can result in increased risk of cardiovascular disease in grandchildren.[94] This is a very powerful concept since it suggests that we are linked to our ancestors not just through our genetic material, but also through their experiences.

Genes and Human Behaviour

The role of the environment on the expression of our genetic material brings to light the impact that life experience has on shaping the developing brain and its subsequent manifestation of the varying human behaviours between individuals. It has been previously assumed that our behaviour was largely a result of genetic predisposition; this is not surprising as genetic research and pharmaceutical research centres have dominated the research arena of changing human behaviour.[95] It is far less popular to critically appraise the impact of societies and cultures on human conduct and action. In a culture fearful of offending varying and highly differing styles of parenting, we are effectively avoiding one of the most important conversations – that is, how to successfully attach with our infants and children.

With our growing knowledge of epigenetics and the limitations of a rigid genetic model (one that states we are at the mercy of our genetics), we can no longer rest easy with the belief that we have endowed our children with a functioning set of 'good behaviour' genes. We are now accountable not only on an individual basis, but also at a cultural and societal level, for the healthy brain development of our children. This, through a natural trajectory, determines the child's capacity to love and to receive love, their moral behaviour, and mental well-being. It is a healing of humanity from the foundations. As Wilhelm Reich asserted, 'civilisation will start on the day when the well-being of newborn babies will prevail over any other consideration.'[96]

What we can definitively state is that the mental health status of the members of our society is suffering, and most concerning are the mental health statistics of our youth.[iv] We have descended into the depths of being the most violent primate, even though we share 99% of our genetic makeup with the bonobo chimpanzee, the most peaceful primate on Earth.[97]

So when did this decline take place, and what has contributed to unhealthy brain development of our youth? This issue is, of course, multifaceted, as environmental influence can be complex, but here I emphasise one of these facets which cannot be ignored; the necessity of healthy mother/infant bonding for the formation of healthy brain development in the child.

[iv] These statistics are discussed in the section 'Our Children, The Canary in the Coal Mine'

James W. Prescott Ph. D, has researched and written comprehensively on this subject and states that 'Extensive scientific research in animals and humans has documented, without question, that mother/infant/child separations (loss of binding/mother love) induces a variety of developmental brain disorders that mediate depression, impulse dyscontrol, chronic stimulus-seeking behaviours and includes self-mutilation, the violence of homicide and suicide and parental violence against offspring.'[98]

If we are to witness a cultural shift and halt the trajectory of human suffering, it is imperative that parents are recognised and honoured as the genetic engineers of our younger generations. Our role is no less important than that. In order for this to take place, support should be prioritised socially and culturally for the primary parents and carers to be present with their children, ideally for the first 5 years of their impressionable life. Other institutionalised settings such as day cares and early preschools should be a last resort.

This can be a very difficult formula to implement in our society. That is why support is necessary at a societal level, resulting in pressure on relevant governmental bodies to recognise the urgent need to support parents of infants and children and to allow them to create healthful loving bonding. This is the way in which humanity can heal.

Epigenetics as Empowerment

Genetic determinism is now a concept that is heavily challenged by epigenetics. We now understand that genes are continually adjusted according to the external environment and our mental response to the environment. We can therefore embrace the changeability of the genome through epigenetics as a source of empowerment. Through our mental state and external environment we are able to manipulate genetic expression – a powerful tool indeed! Just contemplate the benefit to the unborn child if the mother was supported in something as simple as being able to experience elevated emotions rather than stress.

We cannot deny the influence we have over our children's genetic expression, and we can use it as an opportunity to maximise their individual potential. It is also possible to reverse epigenetic markers, another empowering tool for parents wanting to make positive changes for their children. Each child has their own 'bandwidth' of potential based on their genetic makeup, but we have the opportunity to offer them the ability to flourish to the greatest of that potential. Through education and understanding of our ability to control our genetics to a certain degree, future generations can be mindful of their lifestyle choices and therefore strive to positively impact the lives of their own offspring.

Truth 3 Summary

- Epigenetics is the study of how certain influences from the external environment can determine which genes are switched on and off.
- Epigenetics is the link between our heredity and our environment and it can shape our health, personality and behaviour.
- Stress on the mother during pregnancy can result in the generation of epigenetic alternations of the foetal DNA. This can be a powerful influence on the physical and mental health of the foetus post birth and beyond.
- Trans-generational inheritance of epigenetic markers demonstrates how we are not only linked to our ancestors by our DNA by also by their experiences.

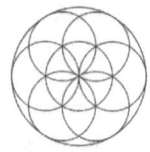

TRUTH FOUR

Monkey See, Monkey Do – Actions Speak Louder Than Words

Mirror Neurons

'The number of permutations and combinations of brain activity exceeds the number of elementary particles in the universe.'[99]

V.S. Ramachandran
Neuroscientist

The complexity of the human brain is endlessly fascinating. As we learn more about its phenomenal characteristics and capabilities, we can parent from a place of knowledge and certainty. An individual's experience of life is a delicate interplay between external events and the mind's interpretation of those experiences. In understanding this, it becomes apparent that the way in which we interact with our children, and the neuronal connections that form as a result, affects the way in which they will interpret this experience we call life.

One intriguing aspect of the human brain is its ability to respond as though it is performing an act, even though the individual is only observing another person doing the particular act. It is an instant connection with another, as one person's behaviour 'mirrors' or triggers neurons in the brain of the other.

Mirror neurons have been described as one of the most important discoveries in neuroscience in the last decade.[100] So what are these brain cells and what is their function?

Mirror neurons are a particular type of cell located in the frontal cortex of the brain. They are exceptional in that they discharge or 'fire' not only when a person performs a specific act, but also when s/he *observes* another individual perform the same act.[101] This system develops in infants before 12 months of age.[102] Mirror neurons are important because they enable rapid learning of complex skills. In addition, they are involved with empathy; the ability to understand what the other person is feeling or thinking from that person's frame of reference.

The brain of the child is able to register the expressions and emotions on our faces faster than they can process what we say – this implies that the child will register our *true underlying* emotions. The most intriguing concept that mirror neurons raise is that we are effectively connected to other human beings by our neurons. The consciousness of each person is connected; we are not discrete from those around us, and the actions and emotions of those around us are firing and wiring our brains and the brains of our children.

In the context of children, the main source of information for their mirror neurons is usually the parents or the primary carers. This is where the beauty of potential arises. As the major role models of our children, we have the exceptional ability to portray those skills and emotions which we want to predominate in the child.

There will always be situations where we do not feel that we have acted in the most ideal way, but we should not feel blame or guilt towards ourselves for this, just more love. We need to always meet ourselves with loving kindness and forgiveness. Through the inner healing that arises from this practice, we can be the most ideal role models for our children.

Empathy

'Be kind, for everyone you meet is fighting a hard battle.'

Plato

As primarily social animals, the function of mirror neurons is very important, as it is key in social interactions, relationships and the experience of empathy and attachment. Empathy is the ability to understand what the other person is feeling or thinking from that person's frame of reference. It can be observed frequently in babies and young children, as they learn by mirroring the facial gestures, language and emotion of those around them. The skill of babies mirroring those around them is the first stage of the development of empathy, or the ability to place oneself in another's position.

Empathy is vital for the experience of sympathy and compassion. Research has explored the neurobiological aspect of empathy, and mirror neurons have been found to be important in the ability to 'feel' the experiences of other people. So why is this response so important? It is crucial because, as social creatures, our survival is dependent upon pro-social behaviours. Empathy guides our behaviour and responses to certain situations.

Empathy also acts as an impetus for morally acceptable behaviour.[103] One could argue that understanding the development of empathy is one of the pillars of a healthy society. Without it social groups could not exist harmoniously. We can see how society deals with those who perpetrate acts that can be described as stemming from a lack of empathy for their victims – we extract and incarcerate them. Recuperation can only take place in the case where the offender experiences remorse, which can only occur on a backdrop of empathy.

Empathy is vital for the development of relationships, self-regulation of emotions and pro-social behaviour. It is the cornerstone of a well-adjusted experience of life. As parents are usually the predominant influence in the early years of a child's development, the child can be seen as reflecting and magnifying who we are, how we feel and what we do. As such, the child is like a barometer of our soul. Children evoke tremendous love, and remarkable frustration, and every emotion between. They make us want to be the best we can, but at times precipitate the eruption of the worst in us. The concept that they are reflecting the aspects of ourselves that we find most challenging is somewhat grating, but on a deeper level most of us realise this is an inconvenient truth. Children have the ability to act as a mirror of such clarity, that at times it can be confronting.

Developing Empathy in the Child

The development of empathy in the child occurs with the completion of the full cycle of connection between the parent/carer and the child. This is the process of interaction and response between the two individuals. Through this process of interaction and connection, as each need of the child is met, we are effectively hardwiring compassion. The child learns through observation and mirroring of behaviours and emotions.

> **The child needs to be loved to show love.**
> **The child needs to be cared for to be caring.**
> **The child needs to be forgiven to demonstrate forgiveness.**
> **The child needs to be respected to show respect.**

This knowledge is incredibly empowering. We are affecting the neuronal hardwiring of our children significantly. It is knowledge that also comes with a great burden. We are largely the reservoir of information that our children tap into to determine how to interact with the world around them. For those children who spend most of their formative years in the company of other influences, the parents should not be surprised if the behaviours and belief set of their child does not closely mirror their own.

Children will use the cues of those in their physical presence as the reservoir of information from which they will fill their knowledge bank of how to interact with the surrounding world. As such, it is imperative that we are comfortable with who is encoding the mirror neurons of our children.

The process of hardwiring compassion in the child's mind by meeting their needs is equivalent to a stone thrown into a pond, with the ripples reaching out to incredible distances. Each child that is provided with the information to encode empathy in their mind will have a ripple effect on those around them, by exuding compassion to those with whom they interact. This would build a new world, one child at a time.

The ability to understand the needs of others also aids the child in being able to recognise their own feelings, and to understand their own emotional needs. The importance of this cannot be overstated, and could be described as being the cornerstone of individual emotional well-being. Without the ability to recognise one's own emotional needs, cracks begin to appear in the emotional relationships that we have with those around us.

There are examples of those beacons of light, who, despite adversity and lack of positive 'mirroring material' in their formative years, have become exceptional examples of human compassion and empathy later in life. The scarcity of opportunities to rapidly mirror emotional intelligence during the formative years does not preclude the ability to develop this as an adult. We are all aware of people who have undergone significant degrees of emotional suffering as children, but have overcome them to be role models for those who have shared similar experiences. The journeys of people who have been through this path are highly inspirational and are an expression of the resilience of human potential. They are a source of enormous power and hope in this world.

Children as Spiritual Teachers

Mirror neurons explain scientifically why the only place we need look to make our child a better person is within ourselves. The ethereal statement that we will affect our children's behaviour and emotional well-being through our own actions is now supported by this knowledge of the connection of our consciousness. We are neurologically entwined with those around us, and this is particularly evident in children. The scientific and spiritual again interlace and dance in harmony.

Many of us have heard the statement that children are among our greatest spiritual teachers. With our understanding of mirror neurons, we begin to realise that the way in which we can moderate and effectively control our children's behaviour is though the moderation of our own behaviour. It becomes a practice of observing the behaviours and emotions in the child and moderating our own behaviours to effect change. There are, of course, situations where a child has genuine developmental and behavioural issues that are not the result of mirror neurons, but rather that of pathological processes within that child. In that situation, this practice has limited effect.

This exercise of observation of the child's behaviours and moderating and changing our own to effect change is not reflective of what most of us practice. This method of changing our own behaviour is a process of exercising less control and not enforcing or dictating prescribed behaviours. Rather, we rely on the child's observation and learning from our own behaviour to precipitate the change.

We need to demonstrate those behaviours and characteristics that we wish to see our children express

This is the ultimate spiritual practice. We are now forced to exercise those characteristics and virtues in the way we live our own life. Trying this for a day is enough to make us realise that this will be a process of dedication and focus! We become accountable for our behaviours and habits. We are limiting our children though our own actions as they struggle to operate beyond the scope of what they witness.

The neurons in the child that are fired and wired together during the most acute stages of development early in life are dependent upon the behaviours and emotions that they observe during this sensitive period. We are not living in isolation – we are not an island; our state of consciousness affects many others, particularly our children. As parents we are now accountable to humanity for raising our level of consciousness so that we can effectively raise the standard of our behaviour.

We have two choices when we witness less than optimal behaviour in our children. Firstly, to react as most of us do, with an unrelenting determination to correct the child. Or secondly, to look within ourselves and determine whether this behaviour is a reflection of some aspect of ourselves that we could improve. In this way, our children are an impetus for our own betterment. They give us reason to reflect on our own consciousness. And for this we should be forever grateful.

Support the Parents of this World

It is acutely important to support mothers and fathers to allow them the best opportunity to display a wholesome and raised expression of themselves. We are all well aware that stress is the perfect environment to lose our focus on expressing a higher version of ourselves. It becomes a collective responsibility to ensure that parents are supported whilst they are parenting young children. Their role should be recognised as one of cosmic importance, as the way in which we influence our children will determine the way in which the world unfolds.

Parenting with Presence

Children provide us with the ideal environment to practise presence and to be more conscious of the present moment. This is one of the most important practises from a spiritual perspective. Children require our aware presence or stillness when interacting with them. We are caught up in a world that is heavily focused on *doing*. Particularly in the west, we have effectively created lifestyles that are an unrelenting series of activities. This can prove to be a challenge when attempting to foster spaciousness within the relationship.

In order for children to be able to practise awareness or stillness, it is necessary that they are able to witness it within those close to them, usually the parents. This is how children can be viewed as our spiritual teachers – they challenge us to remain still and present during some of the most challenging times. It is vital that we provide our children with our attention and our presence, rather than being continually caught up in the myriad of things that we need to accomplish on a daily basis. It is true that it is necessary to get these many things completed, but we must realise that this alone is not enough.

Self-control – A Predictor of Success

The quality that we are exercising when mediating our own behaviour is *self-control*. When we display self-control by regulating our behaviour we are modelling this behaviour for our children. Within the child, wondrous mirror neurons firing away encode this in their neural network as the appropriate way to behave. Demonstrating calmness and presence with the child, at all times, even in times of perceived challenges, equips the child with a neuronal network capable of self-control.

The Dunedin Study[104] is the longest ongoing study of people in the world. It has been following 1000+ subjects since 1972; for over 40 years. In this study, multiple aspects of human health and development have, and continue to be observed, providing detailed information on the accurate predictors for a better life. A particularly interesting aspect of the Dunedin Study is their research into the predictors of *success*. Most interestingly, it was found that the 'capacity to govern ourselves effectively in the face of temptation has profound benefits across every major domain of life functioning'[105] – that is, to exercise self-control. Self-control is the *single most important predictor of success* in children.

This is profound information for a parent wishing to develop self-control in their child, given that self-control is malleable[106] and that IQ and socioeconomic status, the two other predictors of outcomes, are notoriously difficult to influence. The potential we have to alter the trajectory of a child's life based on developing something as simple as self-control is an astounding thought indeed.

Childhood self-control as a predictor of physical health, substance dependence, personal finances, and criminal offending outcomes,[107] makes it a quality well worth developing in the child. As Professor Richie Poulton, Director of the Dunedin study said, the experiences and things that the children do echo down their entire life.[108] Childhood is a foundation for the later years, and the personality of the child that is set in early childhood has lifelong consequences.

What is self-control?

Self-control is the ability to 'delay gratification, control impulses, and modulate emotional expression.'[109] It is the ability to regulate or control behaviour to meet a specific goal. The Dunedin Study showed that children as young as 3 could be tested for their levels of self-control. The method of testing self-control was to put a marshmallow in front of the child and tell them that they would get 2 marshmallows if they were able to resist eating the one in front of them for 15 minutes. As you can imagine, the footage of the example experiment was very entertaining, and the various techniques the children used to resist the temptation were charming.

Methods of developing self-control in the child

Self-control, being the process of delaying gratification, controlling impulses and modulating emotional expression[110], involves the development of each of these aspects of the child. It also requires us as parents and role models to demonstrate this behaviour, even during periods of stress and challenges. There are ways in which we can positively influence the quality of self-control in our children. This could be one of the single most important qualities that we can develop in our children, for from it stem so many opportunities for success later in life.

- Model behaviour
- Provide a relationship of trust
- Encourage initiative
- Reduce stress
- Set boundaries

- Explore reasoning with the child – explain why they should exercise self-control for a particular reason
- Remember the child's brain is still developing and takes many years to fully mature. Exercise compassion regarding their behaviour. They are learning...and it is a long process.

Truth 4 Summary

- Mirror neurons are a type of brain cell that allow rapid learning of complex skills.
- Mirror neurons fire not only when a person performs a particular act, but also when s/he observes another individual performing the same act.
- Children register our underlying emotions mainly through the expressions on our face rather than by what we say.
- Mirror neurons are vital in the development of empathy.
- Children use us as their reservoir of information on how to act and interact with the world around them.
- We need to demonstrate those behaviours and characteristics that we wish to see our children express.
- Self-control is the single most important predictor of success in children.

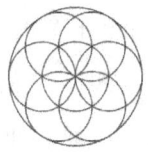

TRUTH FIVE

Our Children are Creative Fountains

The Creative Child

> *'I rest not from my great task!*
> *to open the Eternal Worlds,*
> *to open the immortal Eyes*
> *of Man inwards into the*
> *Worlds of thought:*
> *into Eternity ever expanding*
> *in the Bosom of God,*
> *the Human Imagination.'*
>
> William Blake
> *Jerusalem 5:18-20*

Anyone who has spent time with young children would have noticed their phenomenal ability to play creatively. They appear to be consumed by their inner imagination, oblivious to the constraints of the space around them, or the things within it. It is a beautiful process to observe as they bring their inner imagination and creations into being. They access a world unique to their own mind, and express their world from within with uninhibited wild abandon. It is a common yet wondrous thing to observe, and as adults, it makes us acutely aware of how we have distanced ourselves from and constrained our imaginative and creative world.

Creativity is life itself. Every man-created object before us has first arisen in the human imagination and together with knowledge and motivation, manifested as a physical creation. We are a creative expression of our own thoughts and hopes and aspirations. The power of the human imagination cannot be denied, and this innovative, creative thinking, is what is required for the survival of humanity.

Imagination makes the achievement of our goals possible, and is the gateway to dreams fulfilled. It is an outer manifestation of our inner ingenuity and vision. Creativity is integral to a life fully lived, and our responsibility to nurture and nourish a child's creativity is one of our most important roles as a parent.

The Universe is our Playground

'What you can do or dream you can, begin it. Boldness has genius, power and magic in it.'

Goethe
German Poet, Playwright, Novelist, Scientist

Unleashing the powers of the child's mind

There has been a monumental movement in making adults aware of the limiting effects the mind can potentially have on your life, and methods of overcoming them. What if we were to create a generation of humans who felt empowered rather than limited by the incredible potential of their mental capabilities? We are now becoming aware of the truth that how we *think* and *feel* impacts our personal realities. Numerous authors have illustrated this connection between, mind, body and personal reality. As research grows we are learning more about the overlap of the esoteric and scientific.

What if we did not limit the child's thinking about their abilities? By doing so, are we effectively pruning their neurons with our old limited belief systems? As our external reality is effectively based on the neuronal scaffolding of our belief systems created early in life, can we, through expanding our children's belief set about themselves, push the boundaries of what they are able to experience in their lifetime? I believe this to be possible. By enhancing imagination and creativity, we will exponentially increase the richness of their lives, and therefore the lives of the rest of humanity. This is the groundwork for the emergence of a generation of adults who will meet the future challenges of the world with creative genius.

Creativity

Creativity is the ability to use imagination and prior knowledge to create something new. It springs from a place of novelty and from it is born something of beauty or practical use. Creativity occurs from a place deeper than thought. On a spiritual level creativity can be defined as connecting with a higher consciousness and therefore allowing the flow of this inspiration.

Creativity can be born through the connection with the vaster intelligence. This intelligence is beyond that of the conceptual intelligence with which we are familiar. It is infinitely greater, as it is connection with intuition itself. The ability to connect with this greater consciousness comes through the ability to experience stillness, or presence. There's a Japanese term, "ichigyo-zammai," that means full concentration on a single act. I imagine this as being the origin of creative flow and power. The experience of creativity can be felt like an instant of inspiration, and usually arises from those moments when we are feeling at our peak ability.

All children are born with this strong creative power, and it is necessary to nurture and develop this creativity. Children need to be taught how to apply the conceptual knowledge that they acquire in an imaginative and creative fashion. It is unfortunately the case that the traditional methods of education are based on the conceptual knowledge of facts and information, but at times lack the translation of using this in a creative style.

It is absolutely imperative that our children's creative abilities are nurtured and expanded throughout their education, as it will determine how the human race will cope in the face of adversity in the future. The evolution of creativity will ultimately determine the survival of humanity.

Are we born creative geniuses?

It has now been demonstrated many times that creativity is not a gift with which only a handful of people are endowed at birth.[111] One research study headed by George Land, PhD., an influential speaker, consultant, and general systems scientist, illustrated this. Dr Land founded an institute that researched, consulted and studied the enhancement of creative performance. NASA approached Dr Land with the task of devising a test to identify creative genius as NASA wanted to attract the best minds to work with them.

The test formulated was highly effective, and Dr Land and his fellow researchers became curious about creativity – they wanted to know where it came from and if it is something that is learned. In 1968, the same test, due to its simplicity and effectiveness was applied to 1600 children. The children were tested at 4-5 years old and then tested every 5 years from that point on until they reached 15.

The results were astounding. There was a clear and rapid trending of a reduction in the percentage of children classified as 'creative geniuses' over the 10 years of the longitudinal study. The results were as follows:

	GENIUS CATEGORY FOR IMAGINATION
4-5 YEAR OLDS	98%
10 YEAR OLDS	30%
15 YEAR OLDS	12% (HERE THE STUDY ENDED)
ADULTS (>1 MILLION STUDIED; AVERAGE AGE OF 31)	2%

A staggering 98% of 4-5 year olds in this study were classified as imaginative geniuses. As Dr Land wrote, 'What we concluded is that non-creative behavior is learned."[112] It is astounding that after the schooling experience only 2% of 31 year olds were classified as creative geniuses. What happened to the minds of those children in the interim? It makes me wonder what kind of world we would exist in if the 98% of creative geniuses retained their capacity over a lifetime.

How to light up the creative mind

> *'My contention is that creativity now is as important in education as literacy, and we should treat it with the same status.'*[113]
>
> Sir Ken Robinson
> **British Author, Speaker and Advisor on Education in the Arts**

In order for creativity to flow it is vital to refrain from engaging in 'convergent thinking.' Convergent thinking[v] is characteristic of the analytical, critical mind. When we dive into a creative mindset, we should encourage the child to stay within it and enjoy the creative flow, free from the shackles of the analytical mind. Let the child develop their ability to think of a myriad of solutions to various problems irrespective of how wild and woolly the answers may be. Not only is this enjoyable, but it also nurtures the creative genius with them, and in the process, if we are lucky, we may rediscover the creative genius within ourselves. We can learn from children how to reconnect to the phenomenal power of creativity.

Creativity needs to arise in the land of non-judgment. Most of us know only too well the the fear of being incorrect, and once this emotion rears

---

v   'Convergent thinking' can be contrasted with 'divergent thinking', which is used in the creative thinking process.

its ugly head, flow of creativity is instantly stunted. Keep the emotional environment safe, keep the fight-or-flight brain quiet, and what we will witness is a neuronal dance in vast areas of the mind as the creativity of the child flows. As parents, carers and teachers, our responsibility is to hold this space for the child, because they are the ones who will be responsible for the creative solutions needed in the future.

Creativity is the source of solutions to old problems and becomes the birthplace of society's ability to change, develop and most importantly move forward. The risk of raising children who are unable to connect with their creative powers is dire. The most ominous aspect of a lack of creativity is a generation of children who know only how to conform and stick to rigid patterns.

It will be those children who exist within the realm of creativity as they enter adulthood who will transform and reinvent humankind's existence, and they have the potential to create a new Earth. In order for creativity to blossom, the child must be encouraged, lauded, and given the space to exercise non-conformity. We need to create children who use their beautiful minds to create ideas for change, or we risk stagnating. It is our responsibility to nurture creativity in our youth - our lives depend on it.

The Arts and Their Correlation With Scientific Brilliance

'If you want your children to be intelligent, read them fairy tales. If you want them to be more intelligent, read them more fairy tales.'

Albert Einstein

An interesting study[114] looked at Nobel Prize laureates and their adult arts and crafts avocations. It is well known that Albert Einstein's Theory of Relativity arose from a musical thought, which he experienced due to his love of violin. This study shows that brilliant scientific minds and a love for arts and crafts is a common theme. The research found that Nobel laureates were:

- At least 2 times more likely to be a practicing musician, composer, or conductor
- At least 7 times more likely to be a visual artist, sculptor, or printmaker
- At least 7.5 times more likely to be a woodworker, mechanic, glassblower or interested in electronics
- At least 12 times more likely to write poetry, short stories, plays, essays, novels, or popular books
- At least 22 times more likely to be an amateur actor, dancer, magician or other performer

Santiago Ramon y Cajal, the Spanish father of neuroscience contemplated this relationship when he said 'To he who observes [scientist with artistic hobbies] from afar, it appears as though they are scattering and dissipating their energies, while in reality, they are channelling and strengthening them...The investigator would possess something of this happy combination of attributes: and artistic temperament which impels him to search for, and have the admiration of, the number, beauty and harmony of things.'

Are Intelligence and Creativity Related?

'Art is a vehicle that allows children the expression of a depth and complexity of emotion beyond what their words can convey. Music, art and drama are portals to emotional literacy, a skill we all need to form strong relationships throughout our lives.'[115]

Mary Gordon
Author

The question of whether intelligence and creativity are related has been the subject of empirical research for decades.[116] Intelligence can be described as being 'the ability to learn, understand, and make judgments or have opinions that are based on reason.'[117] This is in contrast to doing something instinctively.

Creativity, on the other hand is the ability to create something new and useful. Current research suggests that intelligence is highly relevant for creativity.[118] The mechanisms by which intelligence cultivates creativity includes 'adoption of smart strategies, high cognitive control and broad knowledge...[and] many creative problems strongly draw on verbal abilities and general knowledge.'[119]

The traditional education system has had a strong focus on 'convergent thinking' that is the thinking of the analytical mind. This is opposed to the 'divergent thinking' utilised in the process of creativity. Although we cannot ignore the importance of convergent thinking, the solutions to problems will arise though the skilful use of divergent thinking. It is within the realms of divergent thinking that we may find resolutions to the conundrums we currently face. Creativity arising from divergent thinking can therefore be seen as nothing less than a super power, and when this is combined with an adaptive intelligence, we will witness a flux of change and problem solving.

Is there a vaster intelligence?

A traditional definition of intelligence can be limited. We are now becoming aware of the various ways in which intelligence can be expressed, rather than the traditional belief that intelligence is a genetic trait that cannot be changed. Howard Gardener is a developmental psychologist known for his theory of multiple intelligences.[120] In his theory, Gardner identified nine different "intelligences" that determine the way we perceive and understand things. They are:

1. Bodily Kinesthetic
2. Interpersonal (communication – verbal and non-verbal)
3. Intrapersonal (self-awareness)
4. Logical-Mathematical
5. Musical
6. Naturalistic
7. Verbal-Linguistic

8. Visual-Spatial
9. Existential[121]

This has implications for the way in which we teach children, as each person has varying strengths and weaknesses in how they understand and process information. The way in which children learn would therefore ideally be by experiencing varied and stimulating environments.

Intelligence of the heart

The concept of 'intelligence of the heart' or 'emotional intelligence' further expands our concept of the various forms of intelligence. In a spiritual context, intelligence can be described as seeing 'the larger whole in which all things are connected.'[122] It is the ability to see all things as part of a much greater picture, rather than as distinct entities. Humanity is reaching a point where it is becoming increasingly important that we see and perceive things as a larger, interconnected experience. We are not isolated in our experiences, and our decisions and actions have much wider implications. An understanding of this vaster intelligence is becoming increasingly pressing for humanity, as we have been thrust into a largely globalised existence where our actions can be much more far reaching than they were historically. No man is an island.

With an understanding of how varied the different intelligences are, we can begin to realise how intelligence becomes dependent on the emotional nurturing of the child.[123] A child who is raised in an environment in which they feel safe will become a child who is confident and trusting of the external environment. This enables them to explore and therefore become the beneficiaries of the unending stimulus around them. As a result, you will have firing and wiring of their neuronal networks, integrating the complex and varied stimulus around them. If the child is exposed to a situation in which they feel fearful and unsafe, it will shut down any desire for them to explore the world around them. As a result the child will never know their full potential, and neither will the world.

The Beauty of Boredom

'When you pay attention to boredom it gets unbelievably interesting'

Jon Kabat-Zinn
American Professor Emeritus of Medicine

We now exist within a society that has a very intense impact on our minds. The ability to be in a constant state of mental stimulation is quite simple to achieve. As this is a relatively new situation in the context of human evolution, it begs the question as to what this constant and unrelenting stream of mental stimulation is doing to the psyche of our young children.

With the important and lifelong implications of neuronal development during the childhood years, parents should reflect on their reflex reactions to children complaining they are bored. It is often expedient to pacify a child with a new toy, electronic forms of entertainment, or perhaps a new book. These are quick ways to fix, short term, what is often a resurfacing and common complaint. Of course, there are times when the above-mentioned sources of entertainment are useful, but we need to assess what our frequent solutions are to this complaint.

Why do children feel bored?

There are various reasons why children may commonly experience boredom. Firstly, it may be the case that the child is accustomed to a highly structured life. When the child becomes dependent on outer direction and structure, and if this is temporarily suspended (school holidays for example), there can be an unease created within the child. Children who are used to someone else directing their activities can almost feel paralysed by the thought of creating their own ideas for enjoyment or play. There is a very strong need for outer direction in these particular children.

There is also the scenario where the child has been involved in an activity that involves too much mental stimulation or 'head' activity. Examples include screen (television, video games, internet), reading, schoolwork or homework. As we know, after such activities our perspective of the world becomes narrowed and contracted. As children innately feel and experience the world predominantly though their bodies, the resulting situation can be a feeling of disconnect. The natural world around them can lose its excitement resulting in the notorious feeling of boredom once these activities are finished.

Boredom as a spring of creativity

> *'If you have young children, give them help, guidance, and protection to the best of your ability, but even more important, give them space - space to be.'*
>
> Eckhart Tolle
Spiritual Teacher, Author

It can be observed that boredom arises essentially from a break from external stimulation. In the case of our modern living, this external stimulation can be incessant and continuous. It is essentially through training our children's minds to be receptive to long hours of stimulation that we negate their ability to cope with the quietness and stillness of their own selves or to observe the subtle beauty of the world around them. It is as though they begin to require external and directed stimulation for an inner feeling of comfort, with an insatiable requirement for amusement.

If we were able to break the overstimulation – boredom cycle that many children are caught in, we would soon observe the magic, splendour and magnificence that can blossom from the quiet of their mind. From a spiritual perspective, the universal consciousness within and all around them can then flow through those wondrous gaps and moments of stillness. We must give our children the opportunities to develop the life-long skills with which to embrace their boredom, and then experience their own stream of consciousness. Let their minds run free, unleashed, unbridled, escaping all constraints and through this they will then truly experience the fluidity of their own minds. No external stimulation could ever match the true beauty of this experience.

Creating an environment for the expression of inner creativity

We must provide an environment in which a child is able to sufficiently express their inner creativity. There are various ways in which we can bolster a child's inner imagination:

- Provide an environment that has various art and craft supplies.
- Easy access to musical instruments.

- Animals for the development of responsibility and of course for the pure joy they bring.
- Various learning materials that are open-ended. Many toys created today preclude the need for any imagination and are therefore not ideal. Try to provide toys that require a degree of imagination, for example things that are not specific in what they could be – blocks that can be a train, car, house, boat etc.
- We as parents have a responsibility to be present and receptive for our children.
- Take the child on a walk in nature to shift their perspective to the physical world around them.
- Encourage the child to go outside and observe the different sounds they can hear, and encourage them to discern the subtleties of nature around them – the different plants, insects etc.

Children are the ones who will be the minds that will create solutions for our future world. We are the parents responsible for providing the environment to shape healthy, creative, and innovative minds. We do not want to be shaping adults that continually need external direction for everything they undertake – paralysed by their own lack of vision and creativity. It is imperative that we are encouraging the development of minds that are able to see the infinite possibilities in the environment around them. It will be these precious moments of insight that will be the seeds that blossom into solutions for the many future challenges.[124]

Truth 5 Summary

- Creativity is the ability to use imagination AND prior knowledge (that is your database of knowledge and experience) to establish something new.
- Creativity arises from a place deeper than thought.
- On a spiritual level creativity can be defined as connecting with a higher consciousness and therefore allowing the flow of inspiration.
- In one study it was found that 98% of 4-5 year olds were classified as imaginative geniuses. This number was reduced to 2% by the time these children were 31 years old. With increasing age the database of knowledge may have increased but is offset by diminishing use of imagination.
- Creativity arises in a non-judgmental environment, and children should be encouraged to exercise divergent thinking.
- Intelligence can be expressed in different ways namely:
    1. Bodily Kinesthetic
    2. Interpersonal (communication – verbal and non-verbal)
    3. Intrapersonal (self-awareness)
    4. Logical-Mathematical
    5. Musical
    6. Naturalistic
    7. Verbal-Linguistic
    8. Visual-Spatial
    9. Existential

- The concept of 'intelligence of the heart' or 'emotional intelligence' further expands our concept of the various forms of intelligence.
- In a spiritual context intelligence can be described as seeing the interconnections of all things as a whole.
- Boredom can act as a springboard to creativity. Allow children the space and time to experience boredom.

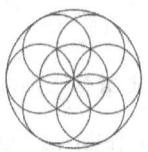

TRUTH SIX

Unconditional Love is a Superpower

Defining Love

To define love remains difficult, with infinite attempts across time to capture its essence through poetry, art, philosophy, spirituality and religion. It spans experiences of parenthood, romantic, sexual, love of the divine, love of the physical world, and of nature. The first experience of love occurs through the maternal. And it is this love that indelibly shapes the individual's experience of love, both in their ability to give and receive it.

The baby's first loving relationship starts with the mother. Within the womb, the baby is awash in the hormones of the mother's emotions. These are the formative signals to the growing foetus regarding what type of environment they will be born into. The development of the foetal brain will wire accordingly. These are the seminal moments that determine how the foetal brain will develop. After birth the babies brain is primed to receive input from the sensorial stimulation from its environment and again wires accordingly.

It is during this formative period that the baby's brain grows and connects as it interprets the world as either hostile or loving. The effects of this first relationship with the mother can potentially have a life-long influence on that individual and the way in which they show and receive love.

How Do I Love Thee?

How do I love thee? Let me count the ways.
I love thee to the depth and breadth and height
My soul can reach, when feeling out of sight
For the ends of being and ideal grace.
I love thee to the level of every day's
Most quiet need, by sun and candlelight.
I love thee freely, as men strive for right;
I love thee purely, as they turn from Praise.
I love with a passion put to use
In my old griefs, and with my childhood's faith.
I love thee with a love I seemed to lose
With my lost saints, I love thee with the breath,
Smiles, tears, of all my life! and, if God choose,
I shall but love thee better after death.

Elizabeth Barrett Browning
Sonnet 43, 1845

Love is a Basic Human Need

> *'If we do not get the sensory stimulation equated with love, bonding and intimacy during the formative periods of brain development, we're going to be impaired, if not crippled in our ability to experience and express this 'language of love' later in life.'*
>
> James W. Prescott, Ph.D.
Brain and Behavioural Neuroscientist, Anthropologist

Love is a fundamental basic human need. It is poetic, that an emotion so difficult to define and describe, can be the primary ingredient of human survival. The fact that the human baby is born as the most vulnerable and dependent of any animal on the planet lifts this requirement for love to unsurpassed levels.

The *way* in which love is expressed to the baby and child is central. Our expression of love towards the child must be in the *language of love* of the child. This was previously a natural instinct of parents, but as we move further away from our instinctual selves, we need to reawaken what previously came intuitively.

This mysterious emotion of love is the vital force and elixir of life. Without it our existence becomes meaningless. As parents, we are endowed with the miraculous ability to encode the brains of our children with the experience of love. This love needs to be abundant; it is impossible to love excessively. This love needs to be all loving and unconditional. It should never be withdrawn and will be a lifelong assurance to these children as they grow, that they will be loved, no matter what circumstances arise in their life. The abundant, unconditional love that we give our children will be the same love that they too will one day give to those entwined in their own life story. Nurturing this ability is the greatest gift that any parent can give their child.

The experiences that are encoded in the baby as love are *body touch, movement* and *smell*.[125] All this is achieved though the activity of attachment with the parent, usually the mother. It occurs during such activities as baby-wearing, breastfeeding, and other actions in which the parent and child are in close proximity. In the case where this sensory stimulation is withdrawn or diminished in the child, the result is incomplete neural development.

The trajectory of children who have had incomplete development of attachment and bonding can, in certain situations, be bleak. It is our responsibility, in light of the current disintegration of the mental health of a drastic number of our youth, to revisit our modern cultural approach to attachment and bonding with our children. There is a responsibility on a social, cultural and political level to assess the effects of effective bonding between parents and their children, and the long-term repercussions on society as a whole.

The results of the withdrawal of love

Many of us are aware of the harrowing examples of children in the past who have been left in certain orphanages or institutions resulting in grave outcomes. It is a stark reminder of the irreplaceable nature of love in the development of children. It has been observed that children in particular orphanages or institutions had serious deprivation to the development of adequate emotional, social and intellectual health. Even in the case where these children were provided with the best medical care, if loving touch and affection were withdrawn, the child deteriorated on every level. In some situations it resulted in the death of the infant.

René Spitz was an Austrian physician and psychoanalyst who observed the different outcomes for infants raised in two settings:

1. In isolated hospital cribs
2. In a prison with their incarcerated mothers

It was Spitz's hypothesis that the poor outcomes in institutions were due to a lack of love. This love deficiency was stifling their development and in some cases resulting in death. His theory was supported by the outcomes of the comparison. Thirty seven percent of the infants kept in the hospital ward devoid of loving touch died, whereas all of the infants who were raised in the prison survived. Those infants who lived in the hospital setting were prone to illness, with psychological, cognitive and behavioural delays and abnormalities. [126] The infants who had remained with their mother, although incarcerated with them, thrived in every way measurable by Spitz.

It is clear from the unfortunate experiences of many infants in certain institutions or orphanages that the result of a deprivation of love is highly detrimental and at worst fatal. Culturally we have come to accept the withdrawal of infants and young children from the parents for a large majority of their waking life. We are the only primates on the planet that have this practice. It is imperative that those infants and children who are experiencing this separation are receiving love and affection from the adults whose care they are in.

Furthermore, we must not forget that our child will be attaching and bonding with the adults or children with whom they are in closest contact. In order to create enduring connections with our children, we need to commit to the process of spending time and attention to re-bond with them on each occasion we are reunited. This commitment to re-bonding is a process that is usually neglected in the time-scarce existence of modern living.

Our Children, the Canary in the Coal Mine

Children do not exist in isolation to the rapidly changing societal shifts. In fact, their psychological health can act as an indicator as to whether the direction we are heading as a society is one that is conducive to well-being. They are like the proverbial canary in the coal mine. It doesn't take much in-depth research on the mental health statistics of children in Australia to raise concern:

- Suicide is the main cause of death of young Australians (aged 15-24), with the number of deaths by suicide being the highest it has been in 10 years.[127]
- Around 1 in 35 young Australians aged 4-17 experience a depressive disorder.[128]
- 1 in 14 young Australians aged 4-17 experienced an anxiety disorder in 2015.[129]
- 1 in 7 young Australians (aged 4-17) experience a mental health condition.[130]

The ominous nature of these statistics should not be ignored. We are failing as a society to nurture the mental health of our children. We need to collectively take ownership of the fact that as a society, we can do things better when it comes to the way we are nurturing the well-being of our children. Mental ill health and suicide are costing Australia up to 180 billion dollars per year.[131] Questioning the foundations upon which the mental health of our citizens is built is an important discussion to have, as it is one facet of the various causative influences that cannot be ignored.

The mental health profile of our most precious cohort indicates raw misalignment and a pinnacle of disconnection. It is imperative that we recognise poor mental health as being one potential outcome of the severed connections in our society and do all we can to re-establish a society that nurtures the brain health of our youth. Although poor mental health can have complex causes, we must do what we can when raising our children to ensure we give them the best possible chance of experiencing normality and freedom from mental illness. After all, these children will be responsible for a time we will not see.

It Takes a Village to Raise a Child

Many parents are floundering in a desperate attempt to juggle the myriad of obligations, and the time and luxury of being attentive and present for their children becomes increasingly challenging. Parents have become victim to a society which does not consider the presence of parents of primary importance. We are struggling to maintain the mental health of our youth and therefore must urgently assess the way in which we are nurturing our young.

This begs the question, which social structure allows for the most effective situation to raise children? The two dominant social structures that humans have existed within are the hunter-gatherer nomadic groups and agricultural societies (horticultural and pastoralism). The hunter-gatherer lifestyle dominated human existence and was a successful system, existing for 90% of human history. Agriculture was established around eleven and a half thousand years ago. By 1500 A.D. most people's food sources came from domesticated sources, although hunter-gatherers still exist today in some parts of the world. Although there are complexities and differences between differing cultures, broadly speaking the establishment of agriculture has enabled humans to exist in a way that is less socially dependent on their communities.

We are no longer required to live closely in communal settings for survival. Today the typical family in western culture is the 'nuclear family.' The effect of this structure is that we are now able to live in relative isolation. This is in contrast to the hunter-gatherer societies that required community cohesion, connection, and support for survival. The aspect of modern living that makes it most appealing, namely the convenience and ease with which we are able to acquire food for survival, has effectively negated the necessity to live in group or community settings.

Without waxing lyrical about the hunter-gatherer lifestyle, we need to acknowledge that human survival occurred within that social model; 90% of human existence was based on this lifestyle. In the context of raising infants and children, we can understand that we evolved to raise them within that social structure - that is one of connection and community. It therefore becomes necessary to observe the approach taken by the hunter-gatherers towards their infants, children and parents, and decide which elements we can successfully adapt to our contemporary existence.

Communal parenting

Baby Homo sapiens, being born prematurely as compared with other mammals, are highly dependent on care, and remain dependent for many years. As Harari explains in his book *Sapiens*, 'This fact has contributed greatly both to humankind's extraordinary social abilities and to its unique social problems. Lone mothers could hardly forage for enough food for their offspring and themselves with needy children in tow. Raising children required constant help from other family members and neighbours.'[132]

This social element of the hunter-gatherer lifestyle is in stark contrast to modern society, in which we can find ourselves isolated unless we make an effort to seek out social interaction. New parents are particularly prone to isolation as the efforts to leave the house with an infant or young child can at times seem monumental. This isolation results in increased stress levels in mothers as many battle at home trying to navigate the difficulties of having a baby.

Stress in the mother naturally impedes bonding with the baby, and the transference of the essential ingredient of life – love - becomes more difficult to bestow - no matter how well-intending the mother. I truly believe it takes a village to raise a child, and our modern existence has moved so far from this model, burdening parents with the sole responsibility of this vastly important role.

The lifestyle of the hunter-gatherer was by no means quiet and relaxed, the female members of the group had many responsibilities that did not stop once children were born. The key difference though is that in the first year of life, the baby was usually carried or worn during these activities.

The women were able to continue with their activities by doing this, with the infant enjoying the benefits of close proximity to the mother and the attachment between parent and child strengthening.

In contrast, modern society separates the mother from her infant if she wants to continue her participation in the workforce. This can cause a deep chasm for many women, as they have a deep desire to participate and continue using their skills, but find it difficult to do so at the expense of bonding with their baby.

The role of raising children was shared amongst women and the younger children in the hunter-gatherer structure. There was a stronger presence of support, as being in close proximity to other women who have been through the process of childbearing and childrearing provides vast knowledge and a sense of security. It is very easy for new mothers in our western culture, through no fault of their own, to become isolated from support, especially if there are no close family or friends who are able to provide time and assistance.

Postpartum depression

The presence of social support during pregnancy, as perceived by new mothers, is a protective factor against the development of postpartum depression.[133] This research emphasises the necessity of societal support for expectant mothers, as the ramifications of a lack of this flows into their parenting experience, which is also the baby's introduction into this world. The support for new mothers gives them a feeling of belonging, purpose, self-worth and importance. This is necessary to bolster the emotional well-being of the mother as she prepares to embark on the journey of human creation.

Although postpartum depression can be a result of many varying factors and combinations of them, we must acknowledge social support as being an important protective factor against it. It is unfortunately the case that many women are not gifted with the social support they need. A society that fails to recognise the emotional well-being of mothers as being profoundly important for the continuation of its stability fails humanity itself.

A mother who is suffering with the darkness of depression, through no fault of her own, struggles to be able to express the fundamental component of life itself – love. Every mother needs to be supported to promote her emotional clarity and emotional well-being. From this position, she can infuse the following generations with abundant, unconditional love, and fertilise the flowering of a conscious younger generation.

Maternal postpartum depression, apart from tainting the mother's experience of motherhood, can have negative effects on the offspring's physical growth. This has been measured. The physical growth of a child of depressed mothers can be stunted, most markedly in the first year of life.[134] It is imperative that a woman experiencing postpartum depression is identified, and supported. In one study it was demonstrated that 'children of mothers who reported symptoms of depression, both postpartum and at follow-up [at 12 years], were at a greater risk of behaviour problems compared to children of women with no depressive symptoms on either occasion.'[135]

Interestingly in the same study it was shown that symptoms of postpartum depression do not in themselves result in an increased risk of behavioural problems in 12 year olds, but ongoing maternal depression does significantly increase this risk. 1 in 7 women in Australia who give birth suffer from postpartum depression.[136] This is not an acceptable statistic. We need to support mothers' emotional health to allow them to thrive postpartum, providing an environment in which the infant and child can flourish physically and mentally, with optimal attachment through love. A society that fails the creators of the next generation is failing mankind itself.

Practicing Unconditional Love Towards Our Children

Unconditional love is the expression of love that honours the divinity within the recipient. It is not dependent on their external behaviour, but is a faith in their inner goodness. Recognising that inner goodness, greater than the person themselves, can sometimes be challenging as it is often obscured by the many layers of conditioned behavioural patterns that we all wear. Unconditional love is a practice of seeing beyond external behaviour to honour that which is within.

Our children are most in need of unconditional love, for it is through experiencing this that they too will uncover their goodness within. The child who observes that those dearest to them have faith in their unchanging and irrefutable goodness will naturally express those values. Over time this will manifest as their prevailing character.

It can be a great challenge to maintain calmness and loving kindness under the typical stress and frustration that parenting can bring. All parents have innumerable examples of times where they have emotionally exploded under the frustration of it all. The challenge for us is to practise expanding the bandwidth within which we are able to maintain emotional stillness. In the same way that we push our boundaries on a physical level to increase our physical well-being, we need to practice discipline and expansion with our emotional growth. Parenting provides one of the most rich opportunities to practice this emotional expansion.

So what does a practical application of unconditional love look like towards our children? There are a number of ways we can practice this superpower so our children grow with the belief system that they are loved, and always will be loved, regardless of where they are at in their dance with life. With this belief, they too will learn to be able to give the same depth of love to those around them.

Love yourself...unconditionally

The ability to love those around you is affected by your ability to love yourself. The deeper the love for yourself, the greater the intensity of the love you can give. First begin to exercise unconditional love towards yourself, and grow in the understanding that you are loved no matter what the circumstance, and you are deserving of love, as we all are:

I am the embodiment of love
I am lovable
I am loving
I am love

Respond to the child

It is imperative to respond to the child when they cry. The culture of allowing children to cry to sleep, cry it out, cry in 'naughty corners', is sending one very clear message to the child – when you cry, no one will respond. This becomes a programmed part of their consciousness. As an adolescent this belief system rears its ugly head as a conviction that 'If I were to reach out for help, no one will be there to listen.' This can be a belief system that carries on throughout life. The messages we are giving our children through our actions are structuring their belief system, for they are in a state of rapid learning about the world around them, how it functions and where they fit in.

Programming is taking place in a child's mind when we adopt practices that involve ignoring a child who is expressing emotion though crying, defiance or other behaviour that we may find challenging. This reinforces the belief that no one will respond when I cry for help. If we do not respond to the child when they cry, we cannot expect that same individual as a teenager or adult to reach out for help when they are in need of emotional support. At no moment should love for the child be withdrawn.

Love the child even when they are at their worst

Loving the child when they are experiencing a behavioural low is a perfect expression of unconditional love. It is also the most challenging for the parent. Most parents are realising that parenting is a spiritual game, where we are stretched to limits that we were unlikely to have experienced previously. Just as adults thrive with loving words and gestures when we reach low points, so do children.

The more challenging the child's behaviour, the more love they require. We need to accept the child for who they are, and also accept the many errors that are made during their path of rapid growth, development and learning. That is the innate difficulty of unconditional love of our children, but the effort put into exercising this gives back a thousand fold as they grow into loving, compassionate, confident young adults.

The Pain of Shame

'The greatest terror a child can have is that it is not loved, and rejection is the hell he fears. I think everyone in the world to a large or small extent has felt rejection. And with rejection comes anger, and with anger comes some kind of crime in revenge for the rejection, and with the crime guilt - and there is the story of mankind.'

John Steinbeck
East of Eden, **1952**

Human beings crave connection; we are hardwired to receive it and when our social connections become threatened the result can be suffering. Love is a part of the vocabulary of connection. We desire to love and to be loved, and through this we create strong connections to those around us. To be deprived of connection harms us psychologically, and physically. The integral nature of connection cannot be ignored, as it is encoded within us as a human requirement.

Infants and children expect connection through love and belonging to a group of people with whom they learn to identify. This has been essential to survival and we are hardwired to require it. In the past, to be ostracised from your tribe was equated with death, and still today we feel an innate need and desire to belong to a group.

Shame is a concept that has been brought to mainstream attention through the enlightening book *Daring Greatly*, by Brené Brown. Brown defines shame as 'the intensely painful feeling or experience of believing that we are flawed and therefore unworthy of love and belonging.'[137] Shaming someone is effectively instilling in them the belief that they, through some innate fault of theirs, are no longer worthy of being a part of the 'tribe'. Severing a person's belief that they are worthy of belonging is harrowing and deeply scarring.

Children are in the process of developing the synapses of connection and love in their sensitive and vulnerable minds. It is a time of acute sensitivity, and a time when the most fundamental and deep-rooted belief systems are established. To harm their sense of love and belonging during this process, can cause a painful trajectory. The vernacular of shame is one where a child is told that they *are* flawed. Such as you *are* a bad child, you *are* frustrating, you *are* a disappointment. It goes to the core of their belief of who they are and scars it. It is distinct from a child being told that they *did something* wrong, which is of course an important part of children learning and creating boundaries.

Shame should never be a method used to control the behaviour of a child. It creates the belief within them that they are imperfect and unable to change positively. The effects are harmful and long lasting. As Brown found in her research, 'shame is highly correlated with addiction, violence, aggression, depression, eating disorders, and bullying. Researchers don't find shame correlated with positive outcomes at all.'[138]

We need to remind ourselves as parents that our children are undergoing a steep learning curve trying to decipher how to navigate the complexities of life. We need to encourage them to take risks and in the process of doing so, expand their experience of life. If we shame children while they are in the process of learning, we effectively clamp their ability to push the boundaries, for they will intuitively do everything to avoid losing the sense of love and belonging that they are hardwired to seek. Children need to *know* that they are loved *no matter what,* and that they are part of their tribe *no matter what.*

Give the Child Space to Feel

A child who is raised to feel unconditional love is given the foundation to live a life of authenticity. By giving the child the space and time to *feel* their emotions, they will grow into an adult who honours their own feelings as valid and meaningful. A child who lives with the belief that they are loved despite their choices will grow and flourish as someone who lives life according to the pull of their heart, rather than by the perceived expectations of those around them. It can take some adults many years to heal from shame and live by their heart's desires. If children are raised to live with the confidence of unconditional love they can live by this basic principle of happiness from the beginning and be a living expression of a divine plan fulfilled.

The Power of a Hug

The expression of love through a hug takes us out of our analytical minds and brings us into the moment. It results in the release of oxytocin, the hormone of love, and promotes feelings of happiness. Interestingly, a study has shown that hugging, or perceived social support, reduced the susceptibility of a person developing the common cold after exposure to the virus. This is consistent with what is called the 'social support stress-buffering hypothesis.' The study concluded that 'those who receive more hugs are somewhat protected from infection and illness-related symptoms.'[139] There is a wonderful power in the hormonal release of a hug. It reduces feelings of stress, it a basic expression of love, and has also been shown to buffer against certain infections. Enjoy the marvellous healing benefits of this experience!

Truth 6 Summary

- Love is a fundamental basic human need.
- We must express our love for our child in the language of the child. For a baby this is touch, movement and smell.
- The deprivation of love towards a baby or child is highly detrimental and has been shown to be fatal in the most bleak examples.
- Mental health statistics of children in Australia highlight the need to nurture the mental health of our children in their formative years to provide them with the best chances of growing to experience normality and freedom from mental illness.
- The presence of social support during pregnancy, as perceived by new mothers, is a protective factor against the development of postpartum depression.
- Unconditional love is the expression of love that honours the divinity within, and is not dependent on the external, but is a faith in an inner goodness of that person - our children are in need of unconditional love.
- At no moment should love for the child be withheld.
- The effects of shaming a child are harmful and long lasting.
- Children need to know that they are loved no matter what, and that they are part of their tribe no matter what.

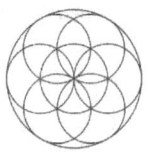

TRUTH SEVEN

You Can't Pour from an Empty Cup

Nurturing the Parent Carer or Role Model

'Yesterday I was clever, so I wanted to change the world. Today I am wise, so I am changing myself.'

Rumi
13th-Century Persian Poet

Every one of us who is fortunate enough to impress upon the life of a child has the reach necessary to change the world. As parents, extended family, and all the support networks of people surrounding children, our impact is no less important than this.

A discussion about how to raise children is incomplete without the realisation that the way we impress upon the child will be equivalent to the way we see and treat ourselves. In this way, parenting is as much about our own path of self-development as it is about attempting to create well-adjusted children.

The way in which we impact upon the child is determined by the way in which we care and uphold ourselves, as it is known that you can't pour from an empty cup. So how do we even begin trying to keep our cup full? The vast majority of us are overrun in our personal and professional lives. Reflecting on possible self-improvement and self-care can easily become neglected.

There are a number of aspects of our self-development that we can use to build a strong foundation from which we can support the growth and development of our children. Without any pursuit of our own self-development, raising well-adjusted children would be an impossibility. Our personal growth and development from a mental, physical and spiritual perspective is intertwined with the whole experience of parenting. We do not exist in isolation. We are inextricably linked to our children.

This is one of the most beautiful aspects of parenting. We are given the impetus to reach for the highest potential of our own growth when we aspire to be the best for our children and ourselves. There is a poetic magnificence to this delicate interplay.

As we grow to love and feel compassion for ourselves, so too will our children learn to love and feel compassion for themselves and those around them. As we learn to forgive ourselves, we teach our children to forgive themselves as they traverse through the highs and lows of life. As we embrace our own imperfections, so will our children learn to love themselves for who they are. For we cannot give that which we do not have. But we receive tenfold that which we have given.

Change

They asked her,

'What is the key to saving the world?'

She answered,

'You. You are the key. Heal yourself, know yourself, make yourself whole and free. Release all limits so that your love can flow unconditionally for yourself and the world, this will open the heaven of your heart completely and it will guide you without fail.'

Yung Pueblo
You Are the Answer

The reasons behind our behaviours and habits are complex. As we all know, it can be extremely difficult to create change in our life. We can drift through day after day in autopilot, as our behaviour and reactions become almost automatic. Anyone who has undertaken this parenting gig before realises that time is not in abundance. We don't have time to sit back and contemplate all the various ways in which we can begin self-improvement. Let's face it; we are lucky to get time to shower, let alone work on the multi-veiled complexity of our personalities. We need a way to fast track filling our cup. We need a way that works on a fundamental level, to create long-standing changes.

The assessment of the world around us is unique to each individual. Every second the brain is faced with a barrage of sensory input, far beyond what our conscious mind would be capable dealing with. The brain has a system to protect itself from this sensory overload. The Reticular Activating

System (RAS)[140] and the thalamus[141] are two areas of the brain that play an important role in this process. They play a key role in what is known as the sensory gating system. It is the nightclub bouncer at the door of the 'Cortex Nightclub.'

The RAS is a net or web-like neuronal network formation located in the brainstem and projects through the thalamus to the cerebral cortex.[142] The RAS is responsible for activating the cerebral cortex and preparing it for the incoming sensory information. The importance of the RAS is so pivotal, that a normal, intact cerebrum is incapable of functioning, consciously and independently, but relies on the information processed through the RAS.[143]

Almost all of the sensory information passes through the thalamus to the cerebral cortex. A major role of the thalamus is to act like a gatekeeper, selecting the sensory-motor information that is sent to the cerebral cortex. The thalamus is controlled by chemicals (or neurotransmitters) released by the brainstem, hypothalamus and cerebral cortex.

We can see that there is a complex interplay between various parts of the brain to determine what information gets our attention and what does not. What is important to understand is that there is sensory input that is ignored to make way for the sensory input that we consider of higher priority. Key things determine whether our brain pays attention to a stimulus or not. These include:

- How prominent or eye-catching it is
- Whether or not we are mentally focused on another task
- Individual ability to pay attention and deal with numerous sensory inputs

- *Expectation – what we consider important based on our prior experiences*

Is believing seeing or is seeing believing?

This begs the question, how does the brain determine what stimuli or data is important and what is to be made redundant? Does this mean that two people observing the same scenario perceive differently? Once you start contemplating the practical meaning of sensory gating, you begin to ponder the deeper meaning of this process. This process literally determines your reality.

Science has commonly held that 'decisions result from the accumulation of samples of evidence informing about the state of the world.'[144] 'Confirmation bias' is the term used to describe the phenomenon whereby choices bias the accumulation of information. This means that the way in which people interpret new evidence is usually based upon their unique previous experiences and choices. Humans are predisposed to seeing information and data that confirms or supports a prior belief.[145] We use this process moment to moment, as it is a mechanism which filters the phenomenal amount of sensory input that needs to be processed, and therefore prevents us from being overwhelmed by TMI (too much information!).

Our existing judgments about a situation actually wire our brain in such a way that we are 'neurally less sensitive' to information that does not confirm our existing belief set.[146] This not only explains the futility of arguing, but also why we are naturally less likely to change our strongly held belief systems. Our brain continually collects data and evidence that reconfirms our history and previous choices. Our sensory gating system is not determining what information is in our best interest, rather it reconfirms what fits snugly with our belief set. Our life can then become like an eternal ride on a Ferris wheel.

Our brain's wiring is effectively creating our outer reality as it searches and selects for data that reconfirms our beliefs. This is our default mode, and to create change we must step beyond our perception, into a place we may not have experienced previously.

Change is a brain game

We are all well aware that attempting to change hurts. In psychological terms this is termed 'cognitive dissonance.' This occurs when a person attempts to hold two or more conflicting beliefs at the same time. This causes mental and physical discomfort. It is much more pleasant to affirm one's assumptions, even when these assumptions are limiting.

Utilising all that we now understand about how we perceive the world around us and how our brain determines what we perceive as important, we can begin to devise methods to create change.

If we are to create long-lasting change, this must occur at a neurological level. We must hardwire a desirable belief structure. As we know, this belief system then informs the gatekeeper of the brain to welcome the stimuli that reinforces this belief set. This is the process of change; this is the process of creating an external reality that reflects the affirmative belief system within your mind, as the mind will see that which confirms its beliefs.

You create change through what you believe and feel

What is your belief set about yourself?

As parents and carers of children, we often question our behaviours and actions. We become more mindful of what we do and say in an effort to carefully protect their minds from our own personal limiting belief set. The first step to change is recognising the limiting beliefs we hold about ourselves. Is it that we are not a capable parent? Is it a victim mentality? Do we believe that we are unable to succeed in life? Am I worthy of love? After all, we understand now why there is always something out there that will reconfirm our belief – it is because our brain is seeking it out.

It is a useful exercise, no matter how uncomfortable, to reflect on what our beliefs are about ourselves.

The secret revealed

Change is a wondrous experience. It demonstrates the human capacity to reach greatness. It is a product of self-control and continued self-correction. We must recognise that we are armed with free will and choice to create in the world around us a reality that matches our desires. This is achieved through the process of firmly held attention. Change at a superficial level is not lasting. We need to delve into the depths of our minds to weed out that which is limiting us and plant the seeds of a belief set from which change will naturally spring. We must arm ourselves with free will in our fight against inertia – this is easier than it sounds.

Taking a step beyond the confines of our brain

Thought and feeling are the creative powers of the universe. And thought and feeling occur through self-control and self-correction. There are no limits to the use of firmly held thought and feeling.

To step beyond the limited confines of our brain's program we must begin by closing our eyes. Then:

- *Visualise* yourself as an embodiment of what you want to become, as the future self you wish to be.
- *Feel* as though this has already taken place.
- *Affirm* with words what is it you are becoming, phrased as though it *already is*:

I am lovable

I am a wonderful parent

I am confident

I am an expression of divine love

I am forgiving of myself and others

I am eternally grateful for my wonderful life

Live with the feeling of being an embodiment of the change you wish for.

High Vibrational Emotions

Love

> 'The teachings on love given by the Buddha are clear, scientific, and applicable... Love, compassion, joy, and equanimity are the very nature of an enlightened person. They are the four aspects of true love within ourselves and within everyone and everything.'
>
> Thich Nhat Hanh
> **Vietnamese Thiền Buddhist Monk and Peace Activist**

Love is one of the highest vibrational emotions. It is also a term that has been adulterated and misused in common vernacular. In that way it has lost its true meaning. Love is being able to see the divinity in the other person, and arises out of a realisation that we are all one. Love springs from presence, and the absence of thought. Once we experience this interconnectedness, love naturally flows and is expressed through emotions such as empathy and compassion. Love is realising that you and the other are one and the same. We must begin with ourselves, and allow love to reside in our body.

Louise Hay in her book *Mirror Work*[147] describes a powerful method for reprogramming your mind to love yourself. It involves using a mirror to look into your own eyes while making positive affirmations and statements of love and affection towards yourself. This is a powerful method of planting the seeds of loving thoughts. Matt Kahn in his book *Whatever Arises Love That*[148] has composed a beautiful healing mantra for making decisions from the heart. This could be a wonderful accompaniment to your mirror work.

I have included below the first paragraph of this healing mantra as I felt the words were very powerful:

> *'I hereby surrender the fate of all my choices*
> *to the highest vibration of love. I allow love in*
> *its purest, most powerful form to fully inhabit*
> *this body, to speak every word, to choose every option,*
> *to orchestrate all behaviors, to maneuver*
> *through each encounter by recognizing each*
> *moment as a chance to speak to others the very*
> *words I've always wanted to hear.'*

Gratitude

'Cultivate the habit of being grateful for every good thing that comes to you, and to give thanks continuously. And because all things have contributed to your advancement, you should include all things in your gratitude.'

Ralph Waldo Emerson
Americal Essayist, Lecturer, Philosopher and Poet

Gratitude is the process of thankful appreciation and acknowledgement of the good in your life. It is the celebration of small victories. This includes both the tangible and the intangible. The process of gratitude focuses our attention on the good in our lives, and in doing so redirects the attention of our brain. It is a perfect example of controlling our brain's filter to recognise the positive, and in doing so we will see more positive in our daily lives.

You can express gratitude for those things around you, or towards your heart or higher self. The emotion of gratitude is of a very high frequency and has the ability to expand the light of your heart and of the world around you. An appreciation of the good that exists in your life, at this very moment, has the effect of attracting and creating abundance.

Science has studied the emotion of gratitude recently, and it has been shown time and time again that people who are habitually more grateful are 'happier than those who are habitually ungrateful; they are less depressed, more satisfied with their lives, have more self-acceptance and have a greater sense of purpose in life. They are also more generous.'[149]

There are various ways to cultivate gratitude in your life; here are a few suggestions to begin the development and expansion of this high frequency emotion[150]:

- Feel/think/express gratitude for the simple things in your life such as a healthy body, sound mind, food in the fridge, clean running water, a roof over your head, a loving family, people who have helped you, Mother Nature, the Universe, the Divine...the list is endless.
- Write notes of thanks to a friend or relative.
- Keep a gratitude journal in which you can write daily the things that you are grateful for.
- If you like to pray, it is a way to express gratitude.
- Meditation is an effective way to focus on the things that you are grateful for. Walking can also be a meditative experience.
- Saying grace before meals is a way to express gratitude daily with your family. It can be done verbally or in reflective silence.

Acceptance

> 'Love only that which happens to you and is spun as the thread of your destiny; for what could be better suited to you?'[51]

Marcus Aurelius
Roman Emperor from 161 to 180 and a Stoic Philosopher

The concept of acceptance, or surrendering to 'what is' liberates you from living in a state of unhappiness. By practicing acceptance we move away from our mental construct of judging what is 'good' or 'bad'. In doing so we exist in a place of equanimity and peace. Acceptance arises from a belief that life is flowing as it should, and that our experiences ultimately direct us to the best outcome, no matter how difficult it may seem at the time. Acceptance needs to be distinguished from inaction. It is still necessary to make decisions, from the heart, and in line with what you feel to be for the greater good of yourself and those around you. Acceptance is the belief that things don't happen *to* you, but they happen *for* you.

Forgiveness

> 'Do the best you can until you know better. Then when you know better, do better.'

Maya Angelou
American Poet, Memoirist and Civil Rights Activist

Forgiveness is a grace that releases us from the suffering that harbouring anger creates. Forgiveness has two aspects, forgiveness of self and forgiveness of others. In this way, it allows you to be released from the emotions of guilt and blame. Forgiveness does not mean that you are allowing the other person to escape from their wrongdoing. Rather, you are releasing yourself from the toxic emotion of blame. In that way it is a healing, uplifting and graceful shift when you practice forgiveness.

An act of self-compassion is forgiveness of self. We all behave according to our level of consciousness at that particular time. The conditioning of our mind manifests as certain behaviour, and while we are on the journey of change, self-compassion is paramount. As our children watch us exercise self-compassion they will also naturally practise this self-love.

Embrace fear

Change evokes fear. It involves shifting to a place we have never known. Humans enjoy change, but not too much! We prefer to exist instead within the Goldilocks zone of change; just the right amount. So many aspects of creating and raising children involve fear. This emotion, if embraced and channelled into appropriate action, can be the precipitant of wonderful change. As we evolve and grow, fear will naturally arise. We should harness its energetic power to propel the growth of our souls, on our infinite path of self-improvement. Without fear we would be unable to gauge when we are stepping beyond our comfort zones.

'It is said that before entering the sea
a river trembles with fear.
She looks back at the path she has traveled,
from the peaks of the mountains,
the long winding road crossing forests and villages.
And in front of her,

she sees an ocean so vast,

that to enter

there seems nothing more than to disappear forever.

But there is no other way.

The river cannot go back.

Nobody can go back.

To go back is impossible in existence.

The river needs to take the risk

of entering the ocean

because only then will fear disappear,

because that's where the river will know

it's not about disappearing into the ocean,

but of becoming the ocean.'

Khalil Gibran
Lebanese-American Writer, Poet and Visual Artist

Raising your vibrational frequency

'Every child begins the world again.'

Henry David Thoreau
American Naturalist, Essayist, Poet, and Philosopher

Through the process of focusing on the emotions of higher vibration we can uplift the energetic frequencies we emit. Love, empathy, gratitude, forgiveness, abundance, compassion, joy, knowledge and empowerment are all emotions that will elevate.

The mother and child are energetically intertwined from the time of conception. By making a conscious effort to develop these high vibration emotions, the mother can uplift the vibration of the child. All we must do is attempt, within our capabilities, to raise our emotional frequency.

While we reside in the space of higher vibrational frequencies our emotional bodies feel light, and the emotions of peace, joy and love are predominant. There is also a sense of clarity and personal power. You will be a shining beacon, lighting up the potential for the future of your children. It is not just the responsibility of the mother to attempt to remain conscious of her emotional state, but also the responsibility of those around to support her. Together we are energetically influencing the outcomes for the child.

Raising children whose natural state is to act in alignment with pure love, combined with the ability to hold steadfast in the honesty of their own being, is the cornerstone of creating a new Earth. In order to achieve this, we must, as carers of the younger generation, choose every word, action and thought with care, as it is through a raised frequency of our own being that we are able to precipitate change in those around us.

As we draw our children into the raised frequency of our own being, we can effectively alter the direction of humanity. We must acknowledge and accept this powerful responsibility as the course of our existence on planet Earth depends upon our children's vibrational default. Our bonds of affection with our children will manifest as an outflow of love and this will propel us into a state of consciousness in which fear, doubt, anger, hatred and greed dissipates. This will then make way for our new Earth.

Finding peace amongst the chaos

> *"Whenever sorrow comes again,*
> *meet it with smiles and laughter,*
> *Saying, 'Oh my Creator, save me from its harm; and do not deprive me*
> *from its good.*
> *Lord, remind me to be thankful,*
> *Let me feel no regret if its benefit passes away.'"*
>
> Rumi
> **13th-century Persian Poet**

Disorder and chaos is a defining feature of parenting. It is heartening to realise that disorder and chaos are also necessary for the evolution of life. A perfect example of this is nature. Within the perceivable disorder and chaos is a beautiful equilibrium, in which there is constant renewal and growth. The chaotic existence of parenting needs to be met with non-resistance, as we walk the tightrope through this period of unstable equilibrium.

Children will be our greatest teachers of patience and acceptance of things as they are in the present moment. They also equip us with the skill of finding the beauty, love, joy and laughter within the chaos. Out of these moments will arise a deeper realisation, of the depth of the present moment. We learn to bless those things that challenge us.

Becoming a parent confronts us with changes in how we perceive ourselves. The construct we had created prior to the role of parent is shaken at its foundations. After all, many of us had been working on this configuration for many years, and then it becomes challenged by the arrival of this little human(s) who demands so much of our time and attention.

This can be a confronting process, but it is also a wonderful opportunity to explore the deeper aspects of ourselves. By embracing the impermanence of our external reality, we can reconnect to the depths of our inner being.

Divine Feminine

> *'Woman is the creator of the universe, the universe is her form; woman is the foundation of the world, she is the true form of the body. In woman is the form of all things, of all that lives and moves in the world. There is no jewel rarer than woman, no condition superior to that of a woman.'*
>
> *Shaktisangama Tantra*

The re-emergence of the divine feminine represents no less than our next evolutionary leap. Men and women both embody a combination of the divine masculine and the divine feminine. Both the divine masculine and feminine are beyond gender and each represents archetypal energies that the whole of human kind embody at different levels. Harmony is uncovered once the middle way of these two energies is achieved.

The archetypal divine feminine represents sensitivity, forgiveness, nurturing, receptivity, expansion, procreation, non-judgment, intuition and compassion. The 'wounded-feminine,' or this energy in excess, manifests as guilt.

The divine masculine embodies the qualities of strength, domination, struggle, striving to achieve approval and self-worth, predation, and protection. The 'wounded masculine' arises in a situation of fear. The divine masculine in its unwounded form can be a highly creative and powerful source.

We can see examples of the masculine and feminine energetic balance throughout various spiritual and religious teachings of the past. This dualism of feminine and masculine is represented in the Yin and Yang energetic concept of Chinese ancient philosophy. Yin being the feminine, is symbolised as receptive and expansive. The Yang energy, on the other hand, is represented as being protective and closed. Yang protects Yin. Yin nurtures Yang. They are both vital for completion of the whole.

Other representations include the Vedic tradition in India, which gives recognition and utmost respect to the female form. The Hindu feminine deity, Saraswati, represents the ideal guru. The name Saraswati translates directly as 'the one who gives the essence of our own Self.' Greek mythology covers the archetypes of the divine feminine, as does Buddhism (Kuan Yin, Tara), and Christianity (Virgin Mary, Our Lady of Guadalupe).

Masculine energy has dominated during the expansion and growth of the western world. This predominant masculine energy has shaped and influenced the things that much of society values today, and many of the archetypal divine feminine qualities became associated with weakness. In the mid 20th century we began to witness a re-emergence of Yin feminine energy with increasing openness and compassion being upheld as valued characteristics.

The divine feminine exemplifies 'being and allowing' whereas the divine masculine represents 'doing and acting.' Most of us would agree that we exist in a state of predominantly masculine energy where our whole existence is experienced in a state of 'doing and acting.' Not only are we existing in this unbalanced state of energy, but we live in a culture that rewards us for doing so. With the imbalance of the feminine and masculine energies, we have also witnessed a lack of compassion towards nature and the resulting environmental challenges we are experiencing today.

We must reverse the subtle but powerful denigration of the divine feminine. True feminism is reclamation of the understanding of the truth of the female body and its divine quality. The divine feminine is the 'real strength' and a re-emergence of this in both men and women, along with a balance with the divine masculine, will result in a seismic shift in consciousness. It is there within us – it is time for women to reclaim the innate knowledge of their immense power and in doing so we will witness a powerful and glorious re-emergence of the divine feminine.

Motherhood and the divine feminine

'Woman knows what true love is; let her not be tempted from her knowledge by the false idols that man has created for her to worship. Woman must stand firm and be true to her own inner nature; to yield to the prevailing false conception of love, of unloving love, is to abdicate her great evolutionary mission to keep human beings true to themselves, to keep them from doing violence to their inner nature, to help them to realize their potentialities for being loving and cooperative. Were women to fail in this task, all hope for the future of humanity would depart from the world.'

Ashley Montagu
The Natural Superiority of Women 1952; **Rev. Ed 1974**

Sakti (Shakti) is a Hindu concept used to describe the primordial cosmic energy - the force that moves through the entire universe. It is the 'Power, energy, capacity, strength, representing the power of consciousness to act.'[152] On the earthly plane, this force is manifested as the divine feminine energy in the female form, and is the power behind creativity and fertility. Through this power, the universe is said to be borne, created and protected. This is one example of a traditional depiction of the magnificent, innate power of the feminine. This feminine energy is so potent, it is life force itself.

For various reasons over time we have witnessed an erosion of confidence or recognition of this power as symbolised in the Hindu concept. This has influenced deeply the way we approach pregnancy, birth and parenting. It is as though over time women have been stripped of their confidence in their own inner 'Sakti', and have a default negative reaction to their own innate ability to access this strength.

Pregnancy, birth and the divine feminine

Through this sensitive process of creation during pregnancy and childbirth, it is wise to shield yourself from negativity or doubt regarding this inherent strength of a woman. Unfortunately, there are many sources of this doubt, but find your tribe, protect and shield your energy, and never doubt the unshakable power of creation that resides within you. Do not fall into the trap of the unending void of self-doubt. Harness your power. Anyone who has witnessed the birth of a child cannot deny the existence of this energy. It is as though this power is from another dimension – like a microcosmic experience of the creation of the universe.

If you doubt your ability to birth your child safely, do not feel negativity or disappointment in yourself. We are, after all, victims of many years of conditioning by a system that thrives on women doubting themselves and their self-worth. The impact this has on the minds of women and their confidence in their bodies is undeniable. When this doubt arises, give it space. It is okay to feel doubt. Meet this emotion with love, and then more love again! And then affirm your ability to birth your child safely, with love.

Birth is a women's rights issue. It is an issue about the right to experience the innate power within. It is a right to birth with dignity, maintaining bodily integrity and autonomy. It is also the right to express our ability to heal the world one birth at a time. Women's birth choices are not to be judged, but it is important that women are helped with reclaiming their ability to access their inner power and faith in their bodies to assist them in achieving the best birth possible for them and their baby.

Bathing our Children in Divinity

Care for our children starts with ourselves. We cannot pour from an empty cup. Our children are intertwined with the energy field and vibrations of the mother and those closest to them. It infuses the child with what is required to live a life of love and fulfillment. Parents who ensure that their own minds, souls and bodies are nourished will bathe their children in the positive emotions they feel. As your cup runneth over, so too will your children be immersed in its goodness.

Truth 7 Summary

- Every one of us who is fortunate enough to impress upon the life of a child has the reach necessary to change the world.
- Key things determine whether our brain pays attention to a stimulus or not. These include:
  - How prominent or eye-catching it is.
  - Whether or not we are mentally focused on another task.
  - Individual ability to pay attention and deal with numerous sensory inputs.
  - *Expectation – what we consider important based on our prior experiences.*
- To step beyond the limited confines of our brain's program we must begin by closing our eyes. Then:
  - *Visualise* yourself as an embodiment of what you want to become, as the future self you wish to be.
  - *Feel* as though this has already taken place.
  - *Affirm* with words what it is that you are becoming, phrased as though you are *already there.*
- The divine masculine and feminine are both beyond gender and represent archetypal energies that each of us embody at different levels at various points in our lives.

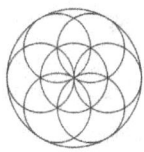

AFTERWORD

'And now here is my secret, a very simple secret: It is only with the heart that one can see rightly; what is essential is invisible to the eye.'

Antoine de Saint-Exupéry
The Little Prince

We are entering a period in which many people are questioning the status quo. On some levels we are witnessing a period of awakening, in which there is a deep and palpable questioning of our purpose and our contribution to our evolving world.

As it is the evolutionary instinct of the universe towards conscious living, many are beginning to reflect on the way in which we experience conception, pregnancy, birth and raising young humans. The recognition that our children hold the keys to our future world makes it clear that the choices we make regarding conception, pregnancy, birth and childhood is a sure method to precipitate change.

Parenting is an incredibly powerful experience, with no finish line. It is the entwined journey of the souls of the parent and child. Contained within this experience is the potential to influence the path of humanity positively. It is no less important than this.

All the information and instinct to do this is already within us. We are designed to be wonderful parents, and every single one of us has this innate capacity. Being reminded of this intrinsic power, and applying the methods to reach it, is an opportunity to raise happy humans and to grow on a personal level.

As early as pre-conception, we are influencing the outcomes of the child. And each step along the way provides multiple opportunities to develop loving, peaceful, compassionate, happy and understanding children. Every time we embrace the opportunity to do this, the world takes one step closer to peace.

Conception, pregnancy, birth, and the early years of childhood are pivotal moments abundant in opportunity to positively impact the child. Although these are acutely sensitive moments, the process of parenting is a continuum, and we can positively influence the child at any point in the process.

When parents experience personal self-development, we witness old habits and limiting beliefs falling away, and something new arising. Through this process we will begin to witness what the true power of love and bonding can do, and this effect will ripple through the entirety of humankind.

As we heighten our parenting experience, we step into the territory of possibility, and we will witness the full potential of humankind unfold. Just like a flower, this unfolding is gradual and takes time. It is a delicate process, but results in perfect beauty. Not only will humanity rejoice in this shift, but also Mother Nature.

Dance of the scientific and spiritual

The process of child creation is an example of perfect interplay between the scientific and the spiritual. We no longer have to make our choices based on the premise of a gut feeling. We now have access to scientific explanations that support our instinctual drive for heart-centred parenting. The more we learn about the child's physiology, brain development and psychological needs, the more we begin to understand the fundamental importance of nurturing the child whole-heartedly.

The gift of parenthood

> *'Let us put our minds together and see what kind of life we can make for our children.'[53]*
>
> Sitting Bull
> **Hunkpapa Lakota Leader**

Our life is a glorious, creative process. It can be a beautiful work of art. Our children bathe and grow in this artwork we are creating. As we mature together to become more aware of what it means to raise children, we create a future of limitless potential.

We have the influence, through a conscious and informed approach to parenting, to change the trajectory of humanity – it is no less important than this. If we want to see an evolution in consciousness on this planet, it is absolutely fundamental that we invest our energy in the creation of a wave of conscious children.

The shifts have the latent capacity to be seismic, and if it is to actualise, the healing effects will echo throughout the future of humankind. We have this possibility within us, as we are gifted with the most powerful tool to affect change, and that is through our children. This is how the world will heal. The moment we realise this is the moment that we can deservedly wear the badge of Homo sapiens – *Wise Man*.

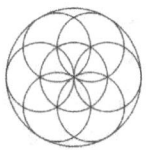

Endnotes

TRUTH ONE

1. Harari, Y., 2011. *Sapiens: A Brief History of Humankind*. London: Vintage, p. 11.
2. Liedloff, J., 2004. *The Continuum Concept*. London: Penguin.
3. Ibid p. 114.
4. Mendizza, M. and Pearce, J., 2004. *Magical Parent, Magical Child*. Berkeley, Calif.: North Atlantic Books, p. 56.
5. Gordon, M., 2009. *Roots Of Empathy*. New York: The Experiment, p. 102.
6. Neufeld, G. and Maté, G., 2014. *Hold On To Your Kids*. New York: Ballantine Books, p. 116
7. Ibid p. 117.
8. Ibid p. 18.
9. I would recommend Neufeld, G. and Maté, G., 2014. *Hold On To Your Kids*. New York: Ballantine Books, for further reading on the subject of attachment.
10. Verny, T., 2019. *Secret Life of the Unborn Child*: Simon & Schuster. As quoted in: *How Much Does An Unborn Child Really Know?* URL: https://biologyofbelief.wordpress.com/2014/07/23/how-much-does-an-unborn-child-really-know/ [Accessed May 2020].

11 Nerburn, K., 1999. *The Wisdom Of The Native Americans*. California: New World Library, p. 99.

12 Verny, T.R. and Weintraub, P., 2003. *Pre-parenting : Nurturing Your Child From Conception*. New York: Simon & Schuster, p. 13.

13 Ackerman, S., 2020. *The Development And Shaping Of The Brain*. URL: https://www.ncbi.nlm.nih.gov/books/NBK234146/ [Accessed May 2020].

14 Verny, T.R. and Weintraub, P., 2003. Pre-parenting : *Nurturing Your Child From Conception*. New York: Simon & Schuster, p. 61. (The other modes of communicating with a foetus are through the senses - touch through the abdomen, sound, and intuitive senses).

15 Ibid p. 9.

16 Olena Babenko, et al. Stress-induced perinatal and transgenerational epigenetic programming of brain development and mental health. *Neuroscience & Biobehavioral Reviews* 2015; 48: 70-91.

17 Lazinski, M.J., Shea, A.K. & Steiner, M. Effects of maternal prenatal stress on offspring development: a commentary. *Arch Womens Ment Health* 2008; 11: 363–375.

18 Verny, T.R. and Weintraub, P., 2003. *Pre-parenting : Nurturing Your Child From Conception*. New York: Simon & Schuster, p. 38.

19 Dr Thomas Verney. Interview in the B*etter Birth 360 World Summit Interview Series 2018*.

20 Odent, M., 2001. *The Scientification Of Love*. London: Free Association Books, p. 15.

21 Rilling JK. The neural and hormonal bases of human parental care. *Neuropsychologia* 2013; Mar; 51(4): 731-47.

22 Miho Nagasawa, et al. Oxytocin and mutual communication in mother-infant bonding. *Front Hum Neurosci*. 2012; 6: 31.

23 Steinbach X. Oxytocin: From a Hormone for Birth to a Social Hormone: The Hormonal Governance of Sociability aka Society. *NTM* 2018 Mar; 26(1): 1-30.

24 Kirkham M, et al. Optimising endorphins. *Pract Midwife* 2012 Nov; 15(10): 33-5.

25 Perinatal Mental Health Consortium (2008). National Action Plan for Perinatal Mental Health 2008–2010, Full Report. Melbourne: Beyond Blue.

26 Silverman ME, et al. The risk factors for postpartum depression: A population-based study. *Depress Anxiety* 2017 Feb; 34(2): 178-187.

27 Ibid

28 Malek A, et al. Human placental transport of oxytocin. *J Maternal Fetal Med* 1996; 5(5): 245-55.

29 Buckley, S., 2006. *Gentle Birth, Gentle Mothering.* Australia: One Moon Press, pp. 123 – 127.

30 Marin Gabriel MA, et al. Intrapartum synthetic oxytocin reduce the expression of primitive reflexes associated with breastfeeding. *Breastfeed Med* 2015 May; 10(4): 209-13.

31 Anderson D. A review of systemic opioids commonly used for labor pain relief. *J Midwifery Womens Health* 2011 May-Jun; 56(3): 222-39.

32 Mark S. Morris, et al. Opioid Modulation of Oxytocin Release. *The Journal of Clinical Pharmacology* 2010 Oct; 50(10):1112-7.

33 Anderson D. A review of systemic opioids commonly used for labor pain relief. *J Midwifery Womens Health* 2011 May-Jun; 56(3): 222-39.

34 Jonas K, et al. Effects of intrapartum oxytocin administration and epidural analgesia on the concentration of plasma oxytocin and prolactin, in response to suckling during the second day postpartum. *Breastfeed Med* 2009 Jun; 4(2): 71-82.

35 Buckley, S., 2006. *Gentle Birth, Gentle Mothering.* Australia: One Moon Press, p. 132.

36 Ibid p. 133.

37 Ibid p. 127.

38 Mercier RJ, Durante JC. Physician and Nurse Perceptions of Gentle Cesarean Birth. *MCN Am J Matern Child Nurs.* 2018; 43(2): 97-104.

39 Wisner, Kirsten MS, RNC, CNS Gentle Cesarean Birth, MCN: *The American Journal of Maternal/Child Nursing* 2016 May/June; 41(3): 186.

40 Stevens J, Schmied V, Burns E, Dahlen H. Immediate or early skin-to-skin contact after a Caesarean section: a review of the literature. *Matern Child Nutr.* 2014; 10(4): 456-473.

41 Guala A, Boscardini L, Visentin R, et al. Skin-to-Skin Contact in Cesarean Birth and Duration of Breastfeeding: A Cohort Study. *Scientific World Journal* 2017; 2017:1940756.

42 Verny, T.R. and Weintraub, P., 2003. *Pre-parenting : Nurturing Your Child From Conception*. New York: Simon & Schuster, p. 212.

43 Odent, M., 2008. *Birth Reborn*. London: Souvenir, p. 26.

44 Verny, T.R. and Weintraub, P., 2003. *Pre-parenting : Nurturing Your Child From Conception*. New York: Simon & Schuster, p. 107.

45 Ibid p. 106.

46 Odent, M., 2012. *Primal Health*. East Sussex: Clairview, p. 60.

47 Moore ER, et al. Early skin-to-skin contact for mothers and their healthy newborn infants. *Cochrane Database Syst Rev.* 2016 Nov 25; 11(11).

48 Bigelow A, et al. Effect of mother/infant skin-to-skin contact on postpartum depressive symptoms and maternal physiological stress. *J Obstet Gynecol Neonatal Nurs.* 2012 May-Jun; 41(3):369-82.

49 Moore ER, et al. Early skin-to-skin contact for mothers and their healthy newborn infants. *Cochrane Database Syst Rev.* 2016 Nov 25; 11(11).

50 Richardson, H.,1997. *Kangaroo Care: Why Does It Work? Midwifery Today*. [online] Midwifery Today. URL: https://midwiferytoday.com/mt-articles/kangaroo-care-work/ [Accessed 26 May 2020].

51 Ferreira M, et al. OC20 - Skin-to-skin contact in the first hour of life. *Nurs Child Young People.* 2016 May 9; 28(4):69-70.

52 Verny, T.R. and Weintraub, P., 2003. *Pre-parenting : Nurturing Your Child From Conception*. New York: Simon & Schuster, p. 104.

53 Qld.gov.au., 2017. *Benefits of breastfeeding*. URL: https://www.qld.gov.au/health/children/babies/breastfeeding/get-started. [Accessed May 2020].

54 World Health Organization statement., 2011. *Exclusive breastfeeding for six months best for babies everywhere*, Geneva: World Health Organization. URL: www.who.int/mediacentre/news/statements/2011/breastfeeding_20110115/en/index.html [Accessed May 2020].

55 Australian Breastfeeding Association., 2011. *Breastfeeding rates in Australia*. URL: https://www.breastfeeding.asn.au/bf-info/

56 www.who.int. (n.d.). *WHO | 10 facts on breastfeeding*. URL: http://www.who.int/features/factfiles/breastfeeding/facts/en/ [Accessed 26 May 2020].

57 Holtzman O, et al. Australian general practitioners' knowledge, attitudes and practices towards breastfeeding. *PLoS One*. 2018 Feb 28; 13(2):e0191854

58 The Australian Breastfeeding Association is a great source of support and information on breastfeeding: URL: https://www.breastfeeding.asn.au

59 McKenna, J.J., Ball, H.L. and Gettler, L.T. Mother–infant cosleeping, breastfeeding and sudden infant death syndrome: What biological anthropology has discovered about normal infant sleep and pediatric sleep medicine. *American Journal of Physical Anthropology* 2007; 134(S45), pp.133–161.

60 cosleeping.nd.edu. (n.d.). *Frequently Asked Questions // Mother-Baby Behavioral Sleep Laboratory // University of Notre Dame*. [online] [Accessed May 2020].

61 James J. McKenna, et al. Mother-Infant Cosleeping, Breastfeeding and Sudden Infant Death Syndrome: What Biological Anthropology Has Discovered About Normal Infant Sleep and Pediatric Sleep Medicine. *Yearbook of Physical Anthropology* 2007; 50:133-161.

62 Ibid

63 Ibid

64 Ibid

65 C Cheng, et al. Supporting Fathering Through Infant Massage. *J Perinat Educ*. 2011 Fall; 20(4): 200–209.

66 Ibid

67 Ibid

68 Field T, et al. Preterm Infant Massage Therapy Research: A Review, *Infant Behav Dev*. 2010 Apr; 33(2): 115-124.

69 Vicente S, et al. Infant massage improves attitudes toward childbearing, maternal satisfaction and pleasure in parenting. *Infant Behav Dev*. 2017 Nov; 49:114-119.

70 O'Higgins M, et al. Postnatal depression and mother and infant outcomes after infant massage. *J Affect Disord*. 2008 Jul;109(1-2):189-92.

71 Tolle, E., 2005. *A New Earth : Awakening To Your Life's Purpose*. UK: Penguin Books, p.127.

TRUTH TWO

72 Gordon, M., 2009. *Roots of Empathy : Changing The World, Child By Child*. NY: The Experiment, p.107.

73 Greenough, W.T., Black, J.E. and Wallace, C.S. Experience and Brain Development. *Child Development* 1987; 58(3): 539.

74 Dennison M, et al. Positive Minds Wire Our Brains for Tough Times. *Australasian Science* 2015 May; 36(4):14-17

75 Gordon, M., 2009. *Roots of Empathy : Changing The World, Child By Child*. NY: The Experiment, p. 66.

76 Ibid p. 67.

77 John W. Whitehead

78 Green C. D. Where did Freud's iceberg metaphor of mind come from? *History of psychology* 2019; 22(4): 369–372.

79 Lipton, B.H., 2016. *The Biology of Belief 10th Anniversary Edition: Unleashing the Power of Consciousness, Matter and Miracles*. Carlsbad, CA: Hay House.

80 Image from: Abhang P.A., et al., 2016. Introduction to EEG - and Speech - Based Emotion Recognition. Elsevier, Chapter 2. URL: https://doi.org/10.1016/B978-0-12-804490-2.00002-6

81 A useful website for understanding paediatric EEG. URL:https://www.learningeeg.com/pediatric

82 Max Planck Institute for Human Cognitive and Brain Sciences, Stephanstrasse 1A, 04103 Leipzig, Germany. As quoted in: Soon, C.S., Brass, M., Heinze, H.-J. and Haynes, J.-D. Unconscious determinants of free decisions in the human brain. *Nature Neuroscience* 2008; 11(5): 543–545.

83 Soon, C.S., Brass, M., Heinze, H.-J. and Haynes, J.-D. Unconscious determinants of free decisions in the human brain. *Nature Neuroscience* 2008; 11(5): 543–545. p. 3.

TRUTH THREE

84 Lipton, B.H., 2016. *The Biology of Belief 10th Anniversary Edition: Unleashing the Power of Consciousness, Matter and Miracles.* Carlsbad, CA: Hay House.

85 Huang, B., Jiang, C. and Zhang, R. Epigenetics: the language of the cell? *Epigenomics* 2014; 6(1): 73–88.

86 Dennison M, et al. Positive Minds Wire Our Brains for Tough Times. *Australasian Science* 2015 May; 36(4):14-17.

87 www.abc.net.au. (2017). How your life could change the cells of your grandkids. [online] URL: http://www.abc.net.au/news/science/2017-04-21/what-does-epigenetics-mean-for-you-and-your-kids/8439548 [Accessed May 2020].

88 Ibid

89 Lipton, B.H., 2016. *The Biology of Belief 10th Anniversary Edition: Unleashing the Power of Consciousness, Matter and Miracles.* Carlsbad, CA: Hay House.

90 Olena Babenko, Igor Kovalchuk, Gerlinde A.S. Metz. Stress-induced perinatal and transgenerational epigenetic programming of brain development and mental health. *Neuroscience & Biobehavioral Reviews* 2015; 48: 70-91.

91 Ibid

92 Rando, O.J. and Simmons, R.A. I'm Eating for Two: Parental Dietary Effects on Offspring Metabolism. *Cell* 2015; 161(1): 93–105.

93 Rando, O.J. Daddy Issues: Paternal Effects on Phenotype. *Cell* 2012; 151(4): 702–708.

94 Rando, O.J. and Simmons, R.A. (2015). I'm Eating for Two: Parental Dietary Effects on Offspring Metabolism. *Cell* 2015; 161(1): 93–105.

95 Prescott, J.W., 2006. How Culture Shapes The Developing Brain And The Future Of Humanity. *Kindred Media*. URL: https://kindredmedia.org/2006/11/how-culture-shapes-the-developing-brain-and-the-future-of-humanity/ [Accessed May 2020].

96 Odent, M., 2011. *Scientification of Love*. Free Association. p. 27.

97 Prescott, J.W., 2006. How Culture Shapes The Developing Brain And The Future Of Humanity. *Kindred Media*. URL: https://kindredmedia.

org/2006/11/how-culture-shapes-the-developing-brain-and-the-future-of-humanity/ [Accessed May 2020].

98   Ibid p. 18.

TRUTH FOUR

99   Ramachandran, V. (2009). *The neurons that shaped civilization.* www.ted.com. URL:https://www.ted.com/talks/vilayanur_ramachandran_the_neurons_that_shaped_civilization [Accessed May 2020].

100 Acharya, S. and Shukla, S. Mirror neurons: Enigma of the metaphysical modular brain. *Journal of Natural Science, Biology and Medicine* 2012; 3(2): 118.

101 Ibid

102 Ibid

103 Decety, J. Dissecting the Neural Mechanisms Mediating Empathy. *Emotion Review* 2011; 3(1): 92–108.

104 Dunedin Multidisciplinary Health & Development Study (Dunedin Study) - Otago.ac.nz. (2016). *The Dunedin Study - Dunedin Multidisciplinary Health & Development Research Unit.* URL: https://dunedinstudy.otago.ac.nz.

105 Duckworth, A.L. The significance of self-control. *Proceedings of the National Academy of Sciences* 2011; 108(7): 2639–2640. p. 2640.

106 Moffitt, T.E. et al. A gradient of childhood self-control predicts health, wealth, and public safety. *Proceedings of the National Academy of Sciences* 2011; 108(7): 2693–2698. p. 2693.

107 Ibid

108 American Public TV (2016). *Predict My Future: The Science of Us preview.* URL: https://www.youtube.com/watch?v=9T7GX3rKAaQ [Accessed May 2020]. As seen on SBS (Aus).

109 Moffitt, T.E. et al. A gradient of childhood self-control predicts health, wealth, and public safety. *Proceedings of the National Academy of Sciences* 2011; 108(7): 2693–2698. p. 2693.

110 Ibid p. 2693.

111 Vint, Larry., 2005. Fresh Thinking Drives Creativity & Innovation. QUICK - Journal of the Queensland Society for Information Technology in Education. Griffith University, Queensland, Australia.

112 George Land and Beth Jarman., 1993. *Breaking Point and Beyond*. San Francisco: Harper Business.

TRUTH FIVE

113 Robinson, K. (2007). *Do Schools Kill Creativity? | Sir Ken Robinson*. URL: https://www.youtube.com/watch?v=iG9CE55wbtY.

114 Root-Bernstein, R. et al. Arts Foster Scientific Success: Avocations of Nobel, National Academy, Royal Society, and Sigma Xi Members. *Journal of Psychology of Science and Technology* 2008; 1(2): 51–63.

115 Gordon, M., 2009. *Roots of Empathy : Changing The World, Child By Child*. NY: The Experiment, p. xix

116 Jauk, E. et al. The relationship between intelligence and creativity: New support for the threshold hypothesis by means of empirical breakpoint detection. *Intelligence* 2013; 41(4): 212–221.

117 Cambridge.org. (2019). *Intelligence | meaning in the Cambridge English Dictionary*. URL: https://dictionary.cambridge.org/dictionary/english/intelligence.

118 Jauk, E. et al. The relationship between intelligence and creativity: New support for the threshold hypothesis by means of empirical breakpoint detection. *Intelligence* 2013; 41(4): 212–221.

119 Ibid

120 Gardner, H. Taking a multiple intelligences (MI) perspective. *Behavioral and Brain Sciences* 2017; 40. E203.

121 Gardner, H.,1999. *Intelligence Reframed: Multiple Intelligences for the 21st Century*. Basic Books

122 Tolle, E., 2005. *A New Earth : Awakening To Your Life's Purpose*. UK: Penguin Books, p. 112.

123 Mendizza, M. and Joseph Chilton Pearce., 2004. *Magical Parent, Magical Child: the art of joyful parenting*. Berkeley, Calif.: North Atlantic Books, p. 48.

124 Williams, L., 2010. *The Heart of Learning - Oak Meadow*. Brattleboro, VT: react-text.

TRUTH SIX

125 Prescott, J.W., 2006. How Culture Shapes The Developing Brain And The Future Of Humanity. Kindred Media. URL: https://kindredmedia.org/2006/11/how-culture-shapes-the-developing-brain-and-the-future-of-humanity/ [Accessed May 2020].

126 Nationalgeographic.com. (2013). *The Orphanage Problem*. URL: https://www.nationalgeographic.com/science/phenomena/2013/07/31/the-orphanage-problem/.

127 3303.0 ABS Causes of Death, Australia, 2012 (2014). Underlying causes of death (Australia) Table 1.3

128 The Mental Health of Children and Adolescents. Report on the second Australian Child and Adolescent Survey of Mental Health and Wellbeing. URL: www.health.gov.au

129 3303.0 ABS Causes of Death, Australia, 2014 (2016). Underlying causes of death (Australia) Tables 11.1 and 11.3

130 The Mental Health of Children and Adolescents. Report on the second Australian Child and Adolescent Survey of Mental Health and Wellbeing. URL: www.health.gov.au

131 McCauley, D. (2019). Mental illness and suicide "costing $500 million a day." *The Sydney Morning Herald*. URL: https://www.smh.com.au/politics/federal/mental-illness-and-suicide-costing-500-million-a-day-20191030-p535r6.html [Accessed May 2020].

132 Harari, Y., 2011. *Sapiens: A Brief History of Humankind*, London: Vintage, p. 11.

133 Tani, F. and Castagna, V. Maternal social support, quality of birth experience, and post-partum depression in primiparous women. *The Journal of Maternal-Fetal & Neonatal Medicine* 2016; 30(6): 689–692.

134 Farías-Antúnez, S., Xavier, M.O. and Santos, I.S.. Effect of maternal postpartum depression on offspring's growth. *Journal of Affective Disorders* 2018; 228: 143–152.

135 Agnafors, S., Sydsjö, G., deKeyser, L. and Svedin, C.G. Symptoms of Depression Postpartum and 12 years Later-Associations to Child Mental Health at 12 years of Age. *Maternal and Child Health Journal* 2012; 17(3): 405–414.

136 Healthdirect.gov.au. (2019). *Postnatal Depression*.URL: https://www.healthdirect.gov.au/postnatal-depression.

137 Brene Brown., 2012. *Daring Greatly : How the Courage to Be Vulnerable Transforms the Way We Live, Love, Parent, and Lead*. Penguin Random House, p. 68.

138 Ibid p. 73.

139 Cohen, S. et al. Does Hugging Provide Stress-Buffering Social Support? A Study of Susceptibility to Upper Respiratory Infection and Illness. *Psychological Science* 2014; 26(2): 135–147.

TRUTH SEVEN

140 Garcia-Rill, E. et al. Arousal and the control of perception and movement. *Current Trends in Neurology* 2016; 10: 53–64.

141 McCormick, D.A. and Bal, T. Sensory gating mechanisms of the thalamus. *Current Opinion in Neurobiology* 1994; 4(4): 550–556.

142 Yeo, S.S. et al. The Ascending Reticular Activating System from Pontine Reticular Formation to the Thalamus in the Human Brain. *Frontiers in Human Neuroscience* 2013; 7.

143 Nolte, J., 1999. *The Human Brain : An Introduction To Its Functional Anatomy*. 4th ed. Philadelphia: Mosby/Elsevier, p. 271.

144 Talluri, B.C. et al. Confirmation Bias through Selective Overweighting of Choice-Consistent Evidence. *Current Biology* 2018; 28(19): 3128-3135.e8.

145 Kappes, A. Confirmation bias in the utilization of others' opinion strength. *Nature Neuroscience* 2019; 23(1): 130–137.

146 Ibid

147 Hay, L.L., 2016. *Mirror Work : 21 Days To Heal Your Life*. Carlsbad: Hay House, Inc.

148 Kahn, M., 2016. *Whatever Arises, Love That : A Love Revolution That Begins With You*. Boulder: Sounds True, p. 65.

149 Sheldrake, R., 2017. *Science and Spiritual Practices*. UK: Coronet, p. 56.

150 Publishing, H.H. (2019). *In Praise of Gratitude*. Harvard Health. URL: https://www.health.harvard.edu/newsletter_article/in-praise-of-gratitude.

151 Aurelius, M. and Hard, R., 2011. *Meditations*. Oxford England ; New York, NY: Oxford University Press, p. 66.

152 B K S Iyengar., 2013. *Light on Pranayama : The Definitive Guide To The Art Of Breathing*. London: Harperthorsons, p. 280.

ENDNOTES - AFTERWORD

153 Nerburn, K., 1999. *The Wisdom Of The Native Americans*. California: New World Library.

Please connect with Dr Karishma Stretton on Social Media.

Karishma can be found at:

www.drkarishmastretton.com.au

@drstretton

Please leave a review on Amazon

www.ingramcontent.com/pod-product-compliance
Lightning Source LLC
Chambersburg PA
CBHW070106120526
44588CB00032B/1185